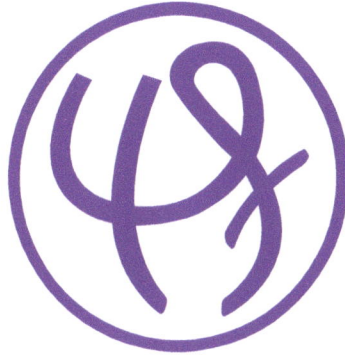

You Are The Horse
&
You Are The Rider

Sara Beaumont-Connop

TheBookStudio

Proudly produced by

TheBookStudio

www.thebookstudio.com.au

Dedication

To my husband, Michael:
He walked the walk and talked the talk.
His artistic spirit is in every nuance of these pages he illustrated or edited.
He has loved this book into Being.

To my Mum, Barbara who let me swing on my first Star,
and to Ola, my Grandmother, Guide and Mentor,
and to Father Brian who always holds us in his heart.

Thanks to all of the people, from babies through children to adolescents;
and all of the grown ups who still brought their own inner children too.
All of you who shared your stories and who gave their permission
for these to be used in forming those stories used therapeutically in this book.

It is also my contribution to you, the Reader;
my hope is that it takes you to wherever you Love to go.

Acknowledgements

There have been a lot of Stable Masters in the writing of this book and the following constitute a beginning of a list: Maryann and Iain Boyd, Bridgette Keenan, Dr Y.C.Lim, Alun and Arlini Evans, Shoshanna Cogan and Shannon Hodges, Dr Mark and Mrs Carol Davis, Rick and Janice Silver, Dr James Allen, Frank Zane, Les and Colleen Mills, Dr Richard Tomlins, Anna Kenna, and Michelle Holyhead.

They have all been inspirational and contributed their wisdom of experiences gathered on this road. Their names will always be up in Highlights for me and I want them to know that in this Universe a book has their names Forever in it!

"This is a brilliantly insightful work exploring the links between body and mind, wellness and dis-ease; both intriguing and innovative, Sara Beaumont-Connop's writing is accompanied by her husband, Michael Beaumont-Connop's sharp and illuminating sketches. This is an absorbing, thoughtful book providing excellent explanations of functional and dysfunctional behaviour packed full with relevant examples from the authors vast professional background and offers cutting edge thinking. This work is rich with story, graphics and an holistic approach for a happier, healthier life, but it's greatest gift is that it offers an accessible roadmap for personal transformation."

Shoshanna Cogan. M.S Counseling. International Training and Consulting. Buffalo NY.

"We change but remain unchanged; we grow but can be unaware of our own wisdom."

SKBC.

"It is a veritable global nomad's guide to the galaxies; all of them; replete with the humour and pragmatism from Down Under. Having worked as a physician for decades with expatriates in overseas settings, there has always been a need for great resource books and here's one you should read and have! The introduction presents the concept of the disparate horse and rider. Through vignettes and well illustrated rich scientific theory this concept grows through the book, culminating in a cleverly integrated function as a "Centaured being."This will join my list of recommended readings. In the waiting room or on the coffee table, it will inspire conversation, introspection and action."

Dr Mark Davis MD. Supervising Physician George Washington Medical Faculty Assoc, Georgetown University, USA. 30 years Expatriate Physician.

"This is such a useful bedside book for everyone who's interested in mental and physical health, both professionals and lay readers!"

Dr Lim Yun Chin MBBS, DPM(UK), M Med(Psych), FAMS, Principal Psychiatrist, Director Raffles Counselling; Psychiatrist Singapore Prisons and Drug Rehab; Visiting Consultant To Institute of Mental Health, Singapore.

"A very readable, very well written impressive book with an intriguing title! The author is a very experienced national and international mental health practitioner. The book skilfully brings together complex and abstruse psychological theories and explains them in a simple understandable form which can then be used by anyone looking to manage change successfully."

Dr Richard Tomlins MB, BB, FRACGP, BEcon, Medicine. Medical Officer DFAT Australia.

"This book is studded with brilliant insights!"

Dr James Allen BA, MS, MD. Senior Advisor, Public Policy and Corporate Responsibility, Chevron. California.

CONTENTS

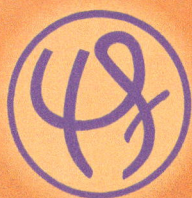

INTRODUCTION

*'The spark of an inspirational idea
can often flare with an offhand remark.'*

The phone rang, quite late in the evening; Crystal as usual was ebullient and hadn't checked the time before dialing. I had just begun mentoring her since her arrival back to Australia for her second attempt at repatriating. Born in NZ and raised in Papua New Guinea for the first 12 years and then Jakarta, Indonesia until she was 25, Crystal was seriously struggling with her new life in Melbourne.

Repatriation is the hardest phase of any expatriate placement and being a third culture kid is the hardest role within that, so Australia, and Melbourne in particular was the very deep end. Complicating that, Crystal was flatting with a young woman that she didn't like or get along with, and who was secretly undermining her. Crystal was attempting to study and become a Naturopath; she was working evenings at a call centre where she had attracted the worst kind of attention from a man who was beginning to look and act more and more like a stalker. Without a vehicle of her own and relying on public transport this particular aspect was dangerously unpleasant.

Work at the call centre had recently deteriorated with spiraling workloads and interpersonal conflicts, and beyond the stalking, Crystal, while ebullient in the face of all of this, had tripped, fallen and cracked a bone in her ankle the evening before, while hurrying home, glancing over shoulder and miss-stepping.

The phone call had Crystal's focus on a desire to change trainings completely, dropping Naturopathy and enrolling immediately in Counselling and Therapy. Crystal was enthusiastically extolling the virtues of a life wherein she could help others, and it was difficult to break into her gallop with an exclamation of: "Hold on Crystal! You're living with someone you really don't like, who is sabotaging your home life, damaging your self-esteem; you have put on weight you don't want and you are not coping with Melbourne's fast lifestyle. You're being stalked; work is full of conflict and stress, you're ambivalent about training as a Naturopath as well as having broken your ankle and getting around on crutches and with all of that, you say you feel like you would really like to help other people as a counsellor! You have got to realise that you are the horse AND you are the rider. It's time to attend to your horse, its lame, injured, highly stressed and in extreme danger; you can't rush off to help others while your own state of being is slowly deteriorating on every level. Your physical self (the allegorical horse) is betraying your intellectual self, one of the first signs of extreme adversity.

Crystal was stunned upon hearing this and for the first time considered the reflected imagery of her separated self, a compartmentalised series of split off parts each almost manageable when considered individually. This is the internal family we carry around within, the child we were, the parents we had, the adult we are, the many messages we receive, all without even being aware they exist.

Crystal is a very resilient and well educated young woman whose apparent ability to manage levels of change was remarkable; however, even she had been unable to see the pitfalls before her. The more she embraced a future complicated with tasks and goals to help others, the louder her own "horse", (child/ physical self) screamed for help. The higher that her anxiety climbed the more she managed it by splitting off bits and pieces of herself, forever imbuing them with positive tasks and roles and becoming less and less cohesive and functional.

"You are the horse and you are the rider!" was a phrase which I uttered spontaneously to Crystal at that time but it was a phrase which expressed much of what I had been developing throughout my own life's quest searching for answers to the riddle of our human experience. The extraordinary manifestation of a being which at the same time has existence physically felt in the world while also inhabiting a consciousness and an even more mysterious unconsciousness. Worlds of thoughts, feelings, psychological energies and metaphysical yearnings which few of us are seemingly able to harness and possess to any degree concurrently and which demands by reason of its manifestation an individual multidimensional analysis and an individual multidimensional solution. Getting to understand that these are internal struggles, discovering where they manifest from, and at what stage of development they represent then integrating them in a healthier holistic expression; was what Crystal would need to do in order to overcome her hurdles and go on to greener pastures.

Have you ever come from a place, such that when you go to find it there's nowhere else quite like it, and there's not; because it was your own childhood?

I was born in the South Island of New Zealand and during my formative years was able to roam wildly in the high country with the sheep and songbirds for companions, in a place where my imagination projected itself onto one of the most beautiful canvases on this planet. My physical world knew few bounds apart from schooling but it was schooling which literally bound me, for when I first entered the tiny, one room school I was told to sit down on a mat and then under a desktop on a chair, pinned like a butterfly to a board! The story my mother tells, is of me, months old and already patrolling the kitchen with her, pulling myself up on her long cotton skirt, tottering forward with first steps, a feat that that floored her!

So the instruction, to sit under a desk, given to a person who had just spent the first five years of their life, mastering the brilliance of their physical body, was nothing short of a declaration of war! These were my first experiences of societies' splitting horse from rider, mind from body; and the next 12 years would follow the same course, an apprenticeship in "desk sitting" with very little movement allowed or encouraged

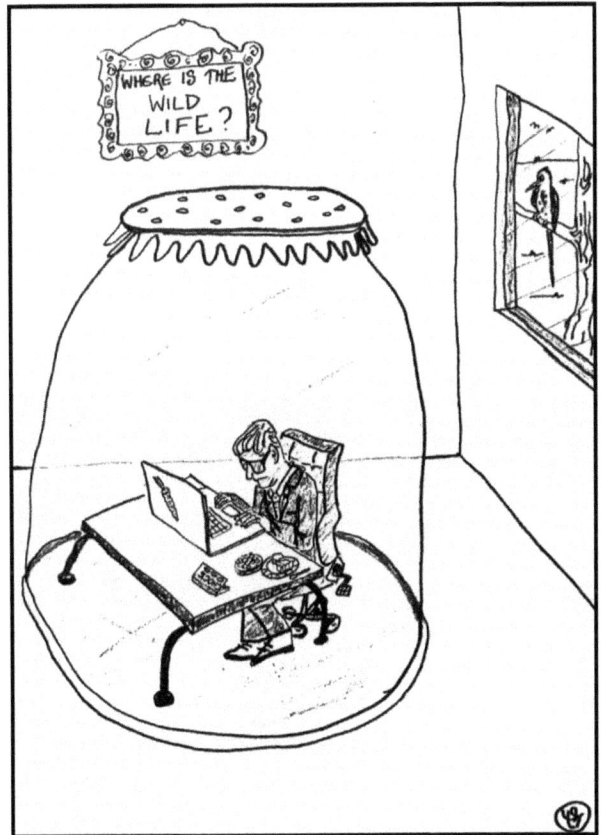

while education was somehow inculcated!

My career has had me moving through various professions beginning with working at a psychiatric hospital, where I witnessed the stunning physical deterioration of young patients within weeks of being admitted. After realising that working with children was my forte I enrolled in Teachers Training College, becoming a senior teacher of junior schools. After being mentored by a psychologist I realised my interest focused more on children with special needs and so I gained further training as a Special Needs Teacher.

I learned that if there is one place in this world that distils the concept of matter over mind and flexibility of spirit it is the challenge of designing Individual educational (on all levels) programmes for children with special needs.

Yelling "Just do It!" is not an option! How do you get a child with cerebral palsy to move in specific ways without complete neural and motor control? I wanted so many answers to so many questions. Confronting the human condition and learning how to enrich the quality of people's lives with whatever obstacles and adversity they faced however daunting it was, would be my work. At the same time as I was working in this field, I was also completing my first degrees in education and psychology and all the while searching for the ideas and concepts behind each training's understandings and offerings in order to answer how I could best facilitate this.

I have always believed in a "practice what you preach philosophy" and an experimental approach to human endeavour, and so, as fortune would have it, in one of those quirky parallel processes, I was invited by a friend to go to a gym with her. Now growing up in the depths of the country where we ran, skipped, jumped and climbed trees with the occasional roll down hills for fun, we did not have access to much sports equipment unless monkey bars and a sugar bag for sack races count so, an actual place, with equipment and weights was a foreign country to me. I was a smallish female, concerned about my weight, of course (weren't we all), but, from good old fashioned stock, people who believed that weights were lifted by males and that women glowed, and didn't sweat.

However, this girl from the country still played bull-rush (a very fast, physical and quite often, violent game!) and knew about number 8 gauge wire (for those of you who don't know; it's fencing wire which can be used for an infinite number of other useful things)! So, daunted but not deterred, I entered that hallowed place: Les Mills Gym, Auckland Central!

I knew I needed to do something physical but something particular, and several days after joining up I found it. It was staring up at me from the cover of a Muscle and Fitness magazine, the face and physique of Rachael McLish, two times female bodybuilding champion in America in the early 1980s. For me this was a revelation, she had an incredible physicality: slender and strong with beautiful symmetry. I wanted that, if I was going to spent time and money in that place that's what I wanted for it, so, time to take my passion and make it happen! It was obvious upon studying the magazine article that Ms McLeish was no Arnold Schwarzenegger and was never going to be; this was the furthest thing from her mind. Health, vitality and beautiful musculature were her only focus!

It took planning, patience, and a dogged determination to stick at it, learn the exercises and start to see the results: muscle toning, waist shrinking and strength improving. However, perhaps the greatest payback were the energy levels I developed, the feeling of a strong body, strong mind, and the ability to take on challenges I never imagined which included completing in the sport and becoming a Les Mills gym instructor, the only woman in the mixed gym, at that time.

The principles of a strong, fit, body and mind helped compel the spirit and life force of this smallish young woman from the smallish green hillock to see that life is full of weights that have to be lifted, full of things that have to be dealt with, things that are not going to go away, and that with a quality of life developed from these principles, I could overcome adversities. Ironically, for me, I had discovered that life's burdens could be lifted in a gym!

Meanwhile I was studying children's behaviors, their many cries for recognition, and in particular, learning to notice how they did it.

Language is not a child's first form of communication, try getting a one year old to tell you all their problems! If your small child needs something, the first sign you will notice is their use of the whole body and sound system in raucous concert! They then refine this to tantrums, kicking, hitting, biting and other symbolic active gestures of dis-ease. In my studies I had viewed many of these behaviours over the years, especially those expressed by troubled children. I wanted to know the meaning of these behaviours and how to help these children to express them without harming themselves or others, to facilitate healing in a holistic way moving them towards a better, healthier and more integrated person.

My questing for these answers then led me to what I thought was the one training which not only subsuming everything I had learned thus far but which then transcended them all, Child and Adolescent Psychotherapy.

It offered the opportunity to analyse and understand the world and mind of the child, to allow the therapist, children and their caregivers the opportunity to go into that world and retrace the steps of trauma and pain through the use of the first language of childhood - active play! Through this methodology comes the most remarkable connections between everyone involved and finally the inner world of the child can be understood.

The symbolic meaning of the child's use of their body in the environment, as understood in play therapy demonstrates the cathartic means of expressing the frustration, anger, pain and suffering we all endure in our childhoods. Many children have smacked their dolly when it's naughty or smashed their blocks apart in anger.

It is the job of the child therapist to put Actions into Words, to connect a child or young person with their feelings and behaviours, which in turn is deciphered for the caregivers, so that the child can be facilitated to move forward into healthier interactions within themselves and their environment.

I gained a place in the post graduate programme of Child and Adolescent Psychotherapy at Otago University NZ where I would graduate 3 years later and begin my practice for the next 20 years.

Part of my training in this work was a 3 year Mother infant observation, which meant that every week for 3 hours I would travel to see the remarkable experience of a child being brought into her family. Seven months before she was born I was there learning about the intra-psychic bonds between mother and foetus and onward through the physical birth and into the years beyond.

Each week I had the privilege of watching a person coming into herself and her environment on every level.

Arguably, after the act of conception, the bringing of that child into the world is the most phenomenal and critical process in life.

We manage to achieve more physical and psychological gains from our conception to the age of 6 years, than we do in the rest of our entire lives!

In this book we will examine some of the theories that form the foundation of these concepts that provide us with the base line of this process: Why it is so important to reconnect with our ability to play, have fun and reengage our physical self on all levels to cope with adversity and journey into overall holistic health.

In chapter One, we will begin to see the relationship and its critical dynamics of attachment with which the mother and child demonstrate and how that determines, in many ways everything the child is able to achieve in the formative years and beyond.

A good example of this is the delight the crawling infant laughingly displays, as it discovers its mother, also delighting in the child's ability to actually master movement for the first time; the discovery that somebody is clapping for us! This "intersubjectivity" between the two is the cornerstone of almost all human progress.

In fact, observations were made during WW2, by John Bowlby, wherein babies who had lost their parents to war, and whom had been evacuated to country manors where every care was made to look after them, actually failed to thrive so badly that they died in wards even though every sustenance was given them. The fact that they did not have the warm, loving attachment relationship with their own caregivers at this time of their lives meant that they were unable to live. Bowlby and his staff, while doing everything desperately to save them noted that the only infants to survive, were those who had formed a special relationship; those who had been designated "favourite" by one or other of the nurses attending them!

This fact, of our utter dependence on a "good enough parent" and its direct relationship to our lifelong psychophysiological development and health is a point of difference so important and so often overlooked, that I make it one of the central theses of this book. The subsequent internalisation that we make of this parent is what enables us as adolescents leaving home and adults in the world, to be successful or not.

Are we able to, later in our own lives, clap for ourselves?

I thought I had the most comprehensive training and experience from which to view our lives, the human condition, and that, with this I would, together with those who chose to work with me, be able to really get to the fundamental issues which have plagued our lives, yet there was something missing! Something really important; the ability to understand and synthesise

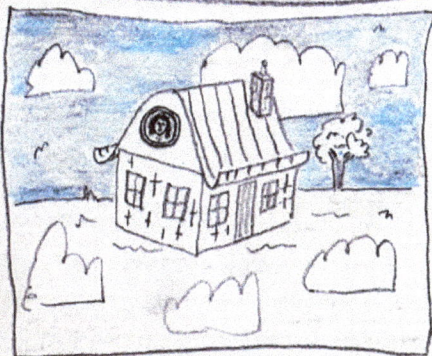

I LIVE INSIDE MY MIND –
INSIDE A BOX LIKE COMPARTMENT

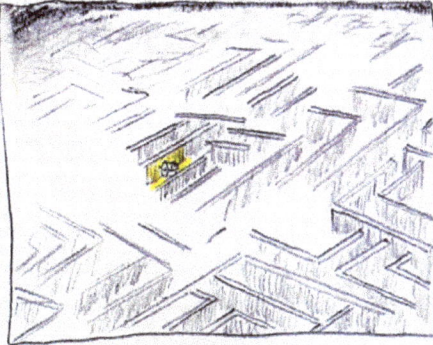

THAT SITS INSIDE
A LONG AND DIZZYING
MAZE . . .

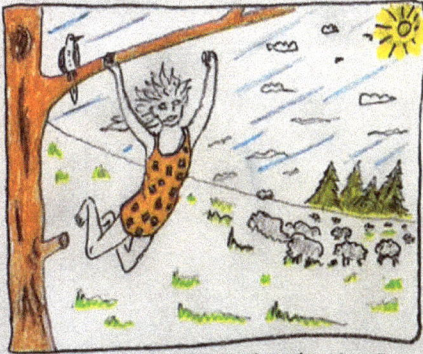

THAT FINDS ITSELF INSIDE A CHILD –
THAT IS BY NATURE, VERY WILD . . .

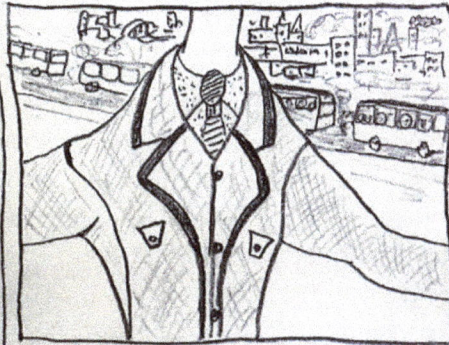

THAT IS LOCKED INSIDE A BODY
THAT IS BLIND TO MY MIND . . .

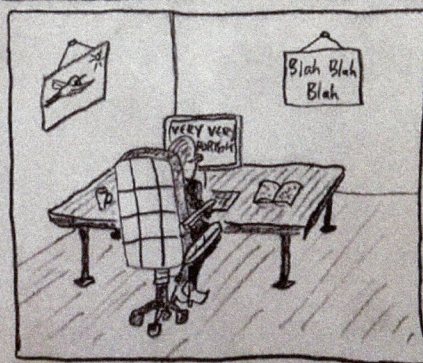

THAT SPENDS IT'S TIME
IN AN ADULT KIND OF WAY . . .

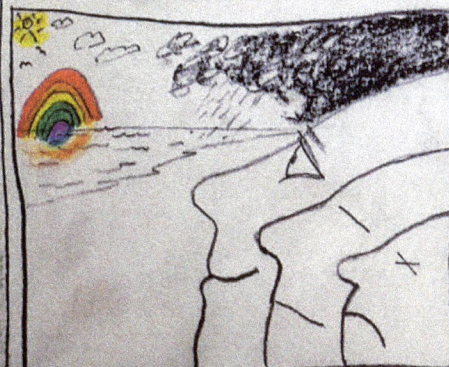

WILL YOU SEE THIS CHILD –
THIS BODY–THIS MIND–
THIS ME ?

the physical and its impact on mental health, and it literally had me out of my seat.

The title of this book is its thesis: We forget at our peril, that at one and the same time, we are both a conscious (and unconscious) being, one which as time goes on, seems to spend more and more of its time inhabiting it's head.

We are also a physical, three dimensional, organic thing, a solid being with a limited lifespan which is dependent on its life to have not only air, water and food but which also only functions optimally, when it is looked after properly.

There is a missing factor in most analyses of function and dysfunction, that of the Horse, the body or soma as it has been known. The child within, the child that is with us always, is subsumed into the horse, and it is this child, our child, with which a good deal of the western world has disengaged, and that will, like Crystal, bring us to our knees if we ignore it, if we only feed it sugar cubes and park it on a chair.

This child, in learning to walk, had a limitless ability to fail, fall and still get up, again and again, for thousands of times…because this child did not know they were failing, sure it hurt when they fell, but they only knew that they were going somewhere... they were growing places!

This book will offer a comprehensive method of assessment with which anyone taking the time to work through, will arrive with a plan to their own individual path of holistic growth.

In order for you to be reading this book right now, please realise that you won the first race, the race to Be You! Of all the hundreds of millions of possible "yous" in the race to fertilise your very own conception, with each possible you, genetically different from every other; it was You who won that race, the Human Race, the greatest race of your life, You, who picked You to be born!

So thrive, read this book and grow places too!

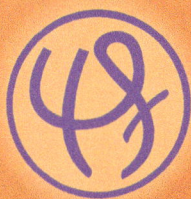

CHAPTER 1

THE PRE-HISTORY OF HORSE AND RIDER

'Freud said we repressed sexuality; Yalom, the creative parts;
I think we repress the entire horse.'

Theory meets Practice

Why are we here, in this particular configuration? A being that has a physical, emotional and psychological reality and as many would say born with a spirit or psyche!

What is the holistic meaning of our lives looked at through the different ages and stages of human development?

The philosophy behind You are the Horse and You are the Rider, comes from the holistic idea that as the Rider we take care for making the choices for our physical manifestation of who we are. I symbolise this physicality as The Horse, the organic mirror image that we present to the world we inhabit. Take a moment to reflect upon what the holistic image is that you project.

Often we are so focused on one aspect of the whole, so split off and lost in our minds that it is difficult to acknowledge that the Body/Horse is sharing the same dimension; remember Crystal!

It is my contention in this book, that the child within does not just die off or go away into the dark recesses of our minds, never to be heard of again. I believe that the child is somehow subsumed within ourselves. The child joins forces through a part of our mind to our body from whence it came, and retains all its physical memories.

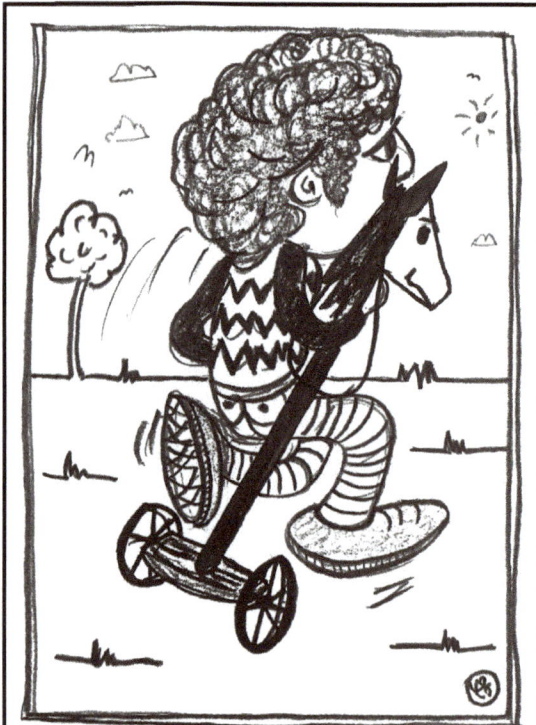

"Sigh, giddy up horse, we've been told to get outside and play!
Let's just show them, let's not have any fun at all!!"

How many levels did we go through to achieve our being? I don't believe that anyone who is reading this book missed out on a developmentally multifaceted, multifunctional series of movements on any of their levels. As children we all attained the physical milestones of crawling, walking, talking, playing, along with the development of all the fine and gross motor functions.

No ordinary child refuses to do those milestones!

The first relationship that developed to sustain the attainment of the goals of existence and growth, was the one created by our caregivers, who held us from the first moment of our conception firmly imprinted in their psyche, imagining our being without even seeing it in reality.

We use this first special relationship; a structure, a framework, to pull ourselves up upon, to look into and see the mirror of self, reflected back over and over again, until we keep part of it in our minds eye (introjection) to sustain and motivate us when the caregiver is absent. I call this part of the self the "Stable Master", the internalized parent, who cares for and make decisions for the Horse/child /physical self.

Finally, the dimension of the adult self is attained as we gain physical and psychological maturity. I have conceptualised this section as the Rider of the Horse. Eventually this Rider will subsume the roles of Stablemaster/Parent as more integrative experiences pass just as the Horse eventually subsumes the roles of Child/Id. The model that ensues is simplified to two balancing systems: Horse and Rider.

It is difficult to be aware that all of these psychological forces are at work within us, vying for pole position as our brain tends to block uncomfortable thoughts and feelings in order to meet the daily environmental conditions of coping with work and relationships from the outside also vying for our attention!

To this end, the ability to choose "Auxiliary Stable masters", for mentoring help and objective support, is often necessary to overcome the impasses life's journey can present to us.

An example of this "auxiliary stable master" might be when the caregiver, responsible for the child's development, commends the child's learning to a teacher, or a physician. They, then become, an extended part of the child's healing in times of sickness or injury, and by doing so, they provide a larger holding environment, which in turn enables the child to learn new skills, to think new thoughts, to safely be supported and lead into his or her own self and the world by way of good motivational or healing role models.

So who are the Auxiliary Stable Masters that mentored my thoughts and theories, what supports these philosophies and working models?

As my studies evolved and took me traveling through the complementary fields of Education, Philosophy, Psychology and Psychotherapy I drew my ideals from a number of models, which makes it a developmentally eclectic approach.

For simplicity I am drawing on Freud's theory and structure of the mind, in order to include some of the basic, yet important psychological constructs, that most of us recognise from everyday speech. Brief descriptions of the model and the terms used will follow. These will assist us to understand the ideas being described and developed later in the book. It is vastly simplified, but as Einstein said: "not too simplified!"

The ID: This is the reservoir of the basic drives and instincts which struggle to rise up and gain expression through our behaviours in the world. These might include hunger, anger, sexuality and many others. This part of the self seeks an immediate reduction of the tension felt within the person without regard for reality. As we come into the world in infancy, we are thought of in this model, as being virtually all id.

It is also thought of acting as the storage repository for inexpressible thought, wishes and fantasies, those which we are uncomfortable thinking about or sharing with others; Freud thought that many of the dreams we have while sleeping came from these tensions and referred to the id most famously as "the unconscious".

The EGO: The self; the "I", which can be understood as the mediator between the person and reality. This is the being that perceives reality and then adapts to it. In Freud's model, the ego is thought of as forming throughout our childhood from the infant id state and achieving maturity through a series of struggles between id drives and superego pressures.

The SUPEREGO: This part of the self is said to give approval or disapproval to the ego activities and punishes or rewards the self. In this model, the superego is thought of as the internalised representations of the parents or caregivers; those people who encouraged or discouraged the child's behaviours by setting boundaries in their various forms.

The superego is pictured above the ego, looking down and watching over what the ego, or self, is getting up to. The id, or unconscious, is pictured underneath the ego, forcing up and into the self's consciousness as many of the desires, instincts and wishes for "tension reduction" that it can!

It is the therapists (Auxiliary stable master) role to uncover the issues that lie, forgotten in the storeroom of the unconscious, but which exist, nevertheless, and bring them into the conscious understanding of the client safely, so that they may better understand how these seemingly forgotten impulses, memories of childhood and hurts are impacting their everyday lives, in often disguised ways, searching for some kind of recognition. These unrecognised indicators (in the life of the client) not only are impeding their growth and sabotaging their lives but are thought to be ways the unconscious parts of us are searching for expression, looking for ways to be able to be recognised and finally be whole with the self, instead of being cast into the unconscious "bin".

Later we will see how some of these processes are acted out in our defence mechanisms.

This is a very simplified version of Freud's theories and is only meant as a framework of application for my own theory and philosophy.

After many years of Freud influencing much of psychology and whilst I was still at Teachers Training College a new book came to my attention, that of "Games People Play" by Eric Berne. It took Freud's Ego, Superego and Id and put them into layman's terms, reinventing Freud's first theories and taking them further into interpersonal relationships.

Eric Berne redefined and renamed the parts of the mind that made up a person's sense of being and simplified them somewhat:

CHILD = ID Berne saw this as a playful and mischievous part of ourselves that did not just fade away into obscurity, but played an active part in interpersonal relationships and personal behaviours.

ADULT = EGO Berne saw this part of the self as that which made the rational, mature decisions, upon which a person based the tasks and directions their lives would take. For example: What career would he or she pursue; when would they start a love relationship?

PARENT = SUPEREGO Berne used the parent to describe this function of the mind and based it on the perceived parenting styles that the child had experienced, he thought, like Freud, that this part of self can be too critical or too permissive with the ID/Child self.

Please refer to Diagram opposite.

The overall sphere is the "psyche" with the individual globes representing id, ego and superego for Freud, or child, adult and parent for Berne.

In his book "Games People Play", Berne suggested that we react to our environment and interact within our relationships from any one of these parts at any moment situationally. This meant that a person could be operating on an adult level at work designing a new building with colleges, operating on a parent level at home putting the children to bed a 7.30pm, and operating on a child level with their partner having an argument about playing on the computer all evening. Behaviour could be explained as originating from the interaction between feelings and thoughts coming from any one or more of these 3 positions, without the person actually realising that this was occurring and the immediate environment they happened to be in. This combination could act as the impetus for any behaviour seen and it was still thought of as being mainly unconsciously acted out.

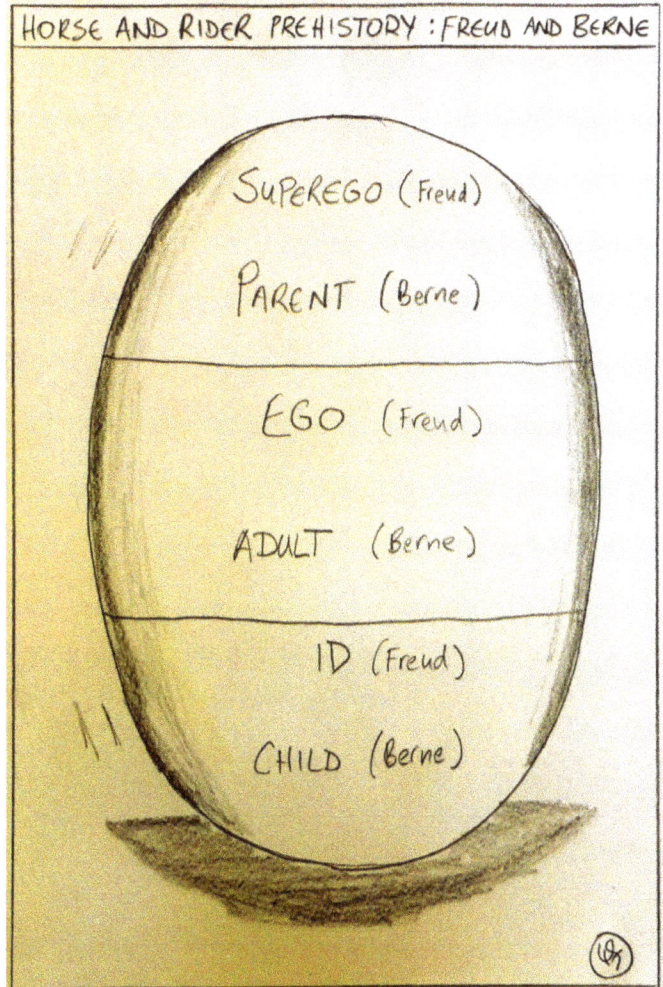

HORSE AND RIDER PREHISTORY : FREUD AND BERNE

SUPEREGO (Freud)

PARENT (Berne)

EGO (Freud)

ADULT (Berne)

ID (Freud)

CHILD (Berne)

This theory became particularly useful when analysing couple and family relating, enabling patterns of behaviour, including intergenerational, to be identified, understood and better integrated forming more mature ways of relating.

Largely missing from Freud and Berne's theories are the basic physical and environmental needs that holistically must be acknowledged as necessary to the physical, psychological and spiritual needs of human existence. Previously people were seen as distinct from their families, communities and environments and their issues identified as being intrapsychic, that is to say, in their heads.

Maslow, a humanistic psychologist, conceived of a hierarchy of these needs, each one being necessarily prior to the following one for adequate growth and depending on that previous need as being met before the next need could be properly addressed.

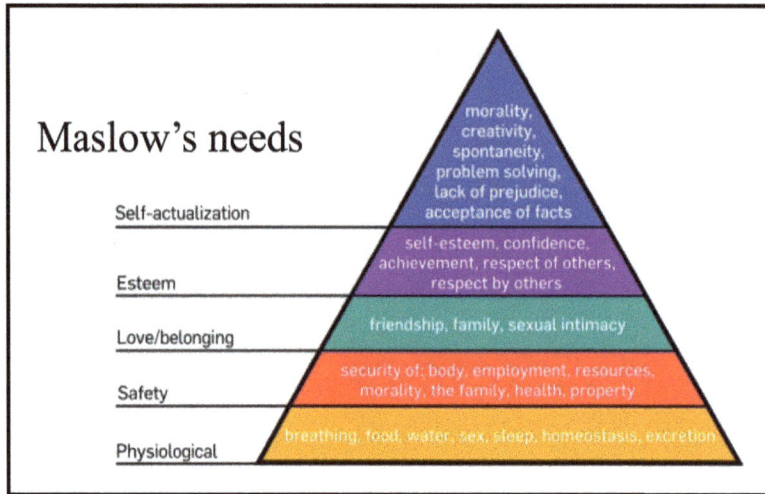

Maslow's needs

- Self-actualization: morality, creativity, spontaneity, problem solving, lack of prejudice, acceptance of facts
- Esteem: self-esteem, confidence, achievement, respect of others, respect by others
- Love/belonging: friendship, family, sexual intimacy
- Safety: security of: body, employment, resources, morality, the family, health, property
- Physiological: breathing, food, water, sex, sleep, homeostasis, excretion

You can't proceed to the next stage fully until you have met the needs of this stage. Maslow placed people into a naturalistic environment and saw their movement towards a full expression of their lives, actualisation, as he called it, as being an evolutionary and normal growth. Psychological health was beginning to be seen in the greater context of holistic health.

I want to add Rollo May, an existential psychologist's statements regarding our existence. He saw people as essentially "free", that they were what they made of themselves, even though there may be "inner conflicts or dynamics" that effected them. People were also seen

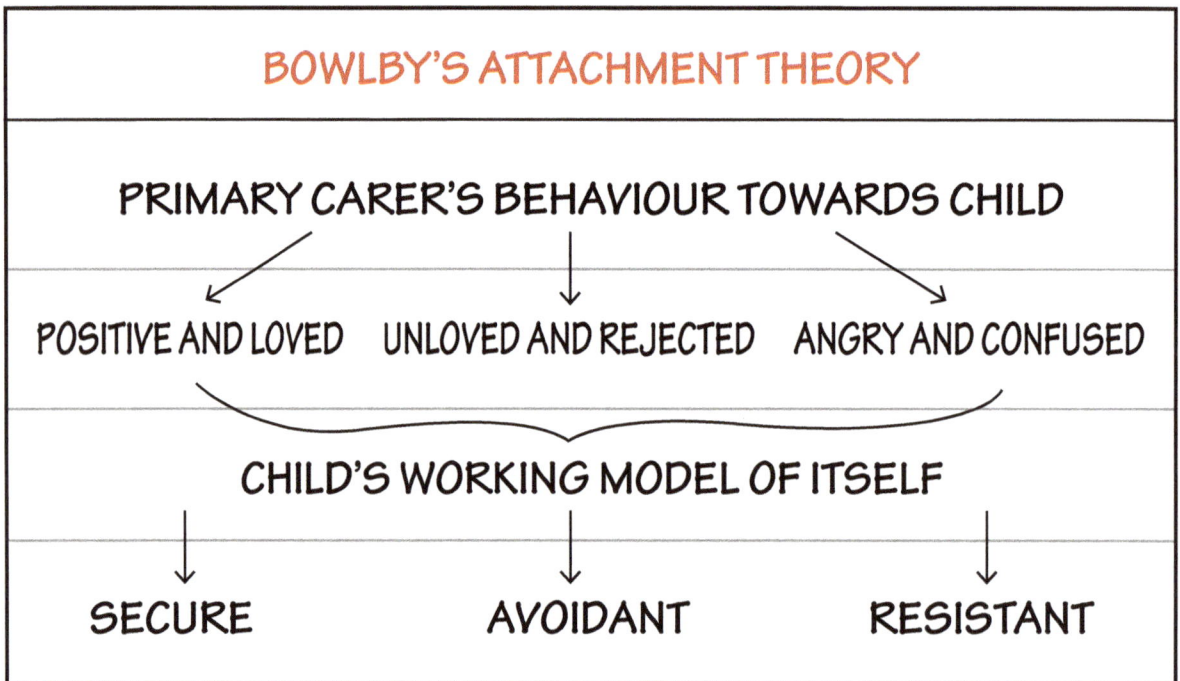

BOWLBY'S ATTACHMENT THEORY

PRIMARY CARER'S BEHAVIOUR TOWARDS CHILD

POSITIVE AND LOVED   UNLOVED AND REJECTED   ANGRY AND CONFUSED

CHILD'S WORKING MODEL OF ITSELF

SECURE   AVOIDANT   RESISTANT

as essentially alone, in that they had to accept ultimate responsibility for their lives and their living; again, even though they lived within relationships with others.

Finally, I am drawing from my own major training Child and Adolescent Psychotherapy. The main concepts come from Winnicott, Mahler and Bowlby who are known as the "attachment theorists". Bowlby's theory that children come into the world biologically ready to attach, similar to Lorenz' studies of geese, allows us to see not only the "imprinting" the child and caregiver relationship provides, but the possible outcomes of this attachment relationship when circumstances are not ideal.

These final few theorists come from a remarkably small but incredibly important field. The study of the psychological birth and subsequent becoming of the child was something virtually and literally unheard of at the time of Freud.

Without this necessarily child-centric understanding, we would be still stuck, trying to find the child by only being able to ask the adult, a little like trying to decide how dinosaurs lived by looking only at their bones!

So we have covered roughly 100 years of psychological thought in a few pages! I am following a particular theme however; the one stretching from Freud through humanistic and existential psychology and culminating with child and adolescent psychotherapy. For those of you reading this book who come from the tradition of psychological thought known originally as "Behaviourism", beginning with Watson and Skinner, leading to cognitive behavioural psychologists and "positive psychologists" like Seligman, I would like to say, that while this book does not follow this tradition, none of the exercises and goals we will be discussing and formulating later would be possible without good behavioural boundaries.

My blue print of "You are the Horse and You are the Rider", is not based in Abnormal Psychology, rather, our ordinary everyday life. I do not want to reinvent the wheel, in fact I am just looking backwards in order to go forward.

My contention is that within every adult there still exists the child and that they can be identified in many different behaviours and feeling states, for example: playing games, buying ourselves presents, and eating favourite foods from childhood.

Not only can this child be felt and act, they can also be heard as a distant voice. The child has become synonymous with our bodies; it has morphed into our physical self, and integrated so completely that it is often unacknowledged.

The child within has become a very important part of a great storage system, one which travels from the conscious experiencing self, to the unconscious reservoir where it is sometimes stored in the physical body, the soma, and if there, it is left just like the lost toy library, where memories are kept, gathering dust, filed, but forgotten, as if by some sort of magic.

The more painful the experiences are of childhood, the deeper they are buried. These are then frequently expressed through the physical body, for instance, the child bullied at school that develops stomach aches to avoid going; the adult stressed at work manifests a cold sore. Sometimes the temper tantrums we have as adults originate from this long buried and needy child who experiences pain, emptiness and rage, but who cannot consciously articulate these feelings, so their body, unconsciously, does it for them. This is a part of ourselves that is crying out for help and it needs acknowledgement and love.

Our mind can operate very much like a library, involving many stories and filled with characters from the past, right up until the present. These characters enact their parts, ascribed to them by our experiences of the situations we passed through with them over each developmental stage of our lives. Experiences such as a parent dying, moving schools or breaking bones are examples of important but traumatic memories while those of winning prizes, learning to successfully ride a bike and being a member of a sports team will be memories filled with joy. The fact is that any drama, good or bad, is an event collated, recorded and stored in our personal library of life (the unconscious mind). It is encoded as a particular memory and it includes all of the people involved with everyone reciting their lines and playing their parts.

When retelling these stories from the past, we are often unaware of how important they are to us, how much they have affected our health and wellness in varying ways both good and bad, and how the weight of carrying and remembering some of them may be putting our back out or giving us a headache.

For example:

A school girl was running for the bus, one winter day after school. She had to catch that bus, the one just swinging into view, heading for the stop. The job she had after school was waiting for her, and they had said that they were not interested in employing late checkout girls. So, she was charging down the hill at full speed, carrying an enormous bag which she had somehow managed to sling over her shoulder, and it was heavy, crammed full to overflowing with every book from every class she had to take.

Just as she approached the final steep descent to where the bus was threatening to pull out from at any second, her feet went flying from under her, the gargantuan bag dragged her down, down onto the slippery, jagged asphalted slope, down into the concrete step, sliding, grazing and slithering to the bottom of the hill, eventuating in rent stockings, a torn uniform, and bloodied and bruised hands, knees and feet. Time stood still!

That woman now can still take out that library book and "be that girl" reading that story 40 years later, with all of the pain, suffering and embarrassed feelings of that adolescent. The girl's horse/body was going where she directed it, but her mind was overwhelmed with stress, she was unable to make good judgement calls regarding her ability to accomplish her goal, that of catching the bus, and combined with the physical weight of the books, the work load she already carried, she quite naturally overbalanced her autonomic nervous system, leading to a complete collapse and a systems failure of her coping mechanisms in the face of the overwhelming odds.

Accidents like this often occur under just such circumstances, as with those which happened in the opening story involving Crystal. Now, when our 50 year old woman experiences similar feelings of stress, the story of running for the bus is retrieved and relived, leaving her vulnerable to sickness and or accidents. These are unusual but exceedingly normal events.

It is important to recognize that within one's self, there exists a "Classified" section of your mind's library; the unconscious. This section can only be opened with a special key and it can only be opened at certain times. One of these times is when the conscious mind is "away", that is, asleep; we dream these stories. The stories here are read over and over as a part of our life story, and they tell us how we coped. Unfortunately, in our example, the character in the story remains a 13 year old girl and the story does not change. The same conditions are still being experienced again and again, just as Jack and Jill, always fall down the same hill, in their nursery rhyme.

Again, please note, that this is not abnormal psychology, it is the ordinary coping and defence mechanisms that we use and it is an essential part of the theory of Horse and Rider.

Understanding the where and how we store our memories, both good and bad; the successes and joys, the failures and hurts which we developed when faced with the opportunities and adversities of our everyday existence is the next step in the book.

Why is it that we don't act upon these things?

As biological organisms our bodies are brilliantly organized into various structures and systems each operating internally, like our veins and arteries, carrying the blood around our body, or our lungs processing the life giving oxygen. We don't see them working, but we know that they are there, doing their jobs, even though they are hidden within us. So too, our mind is operating within us, utilising its different systems, like those of storage and retrieval which are working on several different levels. We don't see them working either, but we do have a multitude of research, psychological, behavioural and biological that says it exists.

In the Model of Horse and Rider (*see diagram on following page*), you will note that the Child has been subsumed into the Horse, the active physical representation of the person. You can see that from the Rider's perspective, it might sometimes difficult to acknowledge the Horse's active role in their wellbeing, however the foundation of the circle is the physical self, from which the Horse emanates, the Horse, whose existence is the biologically given.

Again, childhood is not optional! We all have to have a childhood and we all have memories, feelings and experiences from that stage of our development.

The Child's basic imperative is to "grow up!" No one gets the opportunity, in the normal sense we are using, to refuse this task. Changing diapers, for the ordinary person at the age of 30 is either unfortunate or is in the realm of abnormal psychology.

We frequently think that "we" are essentially only a thinking being (Rene Descartes: "I think, therefore I am"); and by virtue of this we are in denial with regard to our "Horse", our physical being and it's systems.

As the Rider we are also frequently in a similar sense of denial with regard to the fact that we were children and we pretend that stage of our being is "now extinct" or over. What is it that we have managed to do internally to overcome these facts, and how was it that we even got to grow up, given there were so many competing feelings and experiences which we had to convert into various responses then memories, not to mention the myriad of skills and tasks to learn?

What has happened to all this information?

ADULT OR EGO
INTELLECT MINDFULLNESS
SELF-OBSERVING EGO
MAPS FUTURE, PLANS PATHS
CHOOSES, USES HIGHER
DEFENCES, HUMOUR

SUPER-EGO OR STABLEMASTER
EMPATHY FOR SELF AND OTHER
CAPACITY FOR CONCERN
CARRIES FAMILIES UNCONSCIOUS INTROJECT
INTERPRETS CHILD'S NEEDS
CAN BE PUNITIVE
SENSE OF SOCIETY

RIDER

HORSE

SOMA OR ID
PHYSICAL ACHIEVEMENTS, WALKING
STORAGE BIN STRESS
EATING, IN-THE MOMENT
FINE AND GROSS MOTOR SKILLS

GOOD VS BAD
SPLITTING PART-OBJECTS
EMOTIONS AND ATTACHMENTS
SPONTANEOUS PLAY, JOY AND CREATIVITY
STORAGE OF CHILD'S UNCONSCIOUS HURTS
CHILD

DEVELOPMENTAL MODEL OF HORSE AND RIDER

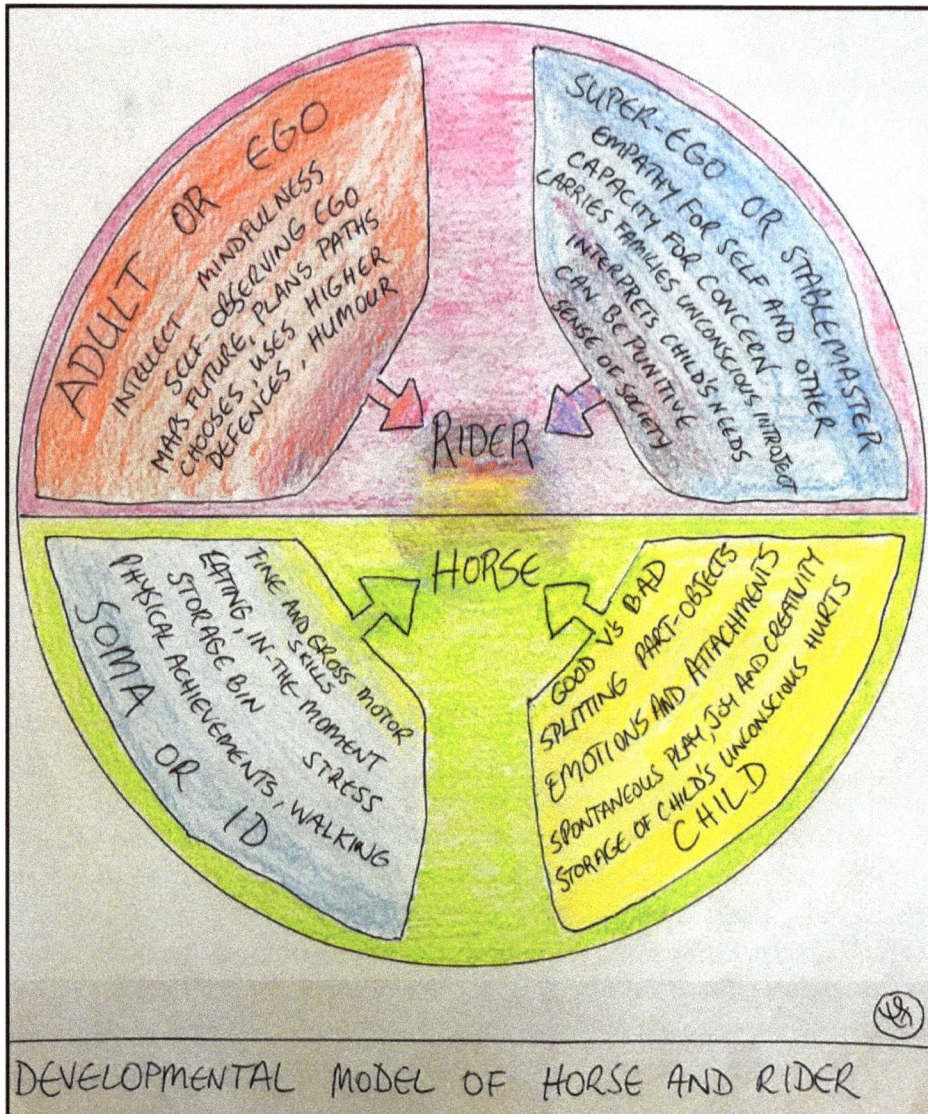

Why doesn't this information deluge overwhelm the development and growth of these two systems, mind and body?

Here we are beginning to see the first traces of an answer to this chapter's initial question: Why are we in this configuration?

The system we inhabit is in fact, one and the same, but somehow strangely joined. We have within us something I like to call the Pony Express system; the first beginnings of that internal library. The Pony Express operates by taking some messages and storing them in the saddlebags of the Horse, the other messages are carried by the Rider. When the Rider's bag gets too heavy and overwhelming the Horse is always there to carry it.

This system has a duality of nature that we are aware of even though we might not know exactly how it is working: the Classified Section. As previously discussed, Freud saw this part of us as corresponding to our instinctual drives, the good the bad and the ugly. Along with these drives, urges and instincts, the environment also impinges upon the person, creating the experiences being converted into the messages carried in these dual natured bags. They might include the traumas, the experiences of being parented, for better or for worse and the interactions with the community at large. The Pony Express carries all of these early messages and stories allowing the child to run and jump the milestones of growing up.

Our "mindbody", has been and is interacting on every level of our being in a multiplicity of ways and for example, the very movements we had to practice and master as infants, over thousands of times, we "forget", as they have become "second nature", imagine every time you had to walk somewhere you had to remember how to walk!

These saddlebags which carry the overload messages, the traumas including the thousand falls, the millions upon millions of moments which we all experience as we grow and which have all been sorted by the Pony Express, act in exactly the same way as Mary Poppins' carpetbag, or Hermione's handbag out of Harry Potter; a magic container that has an infinite capacity and secret compartments within it, carried everywhere and dipped into when necessary. In a short while we will see how the bags operate discriminating which section of the library books are sorted to.

The ability to be objectively aware of one's own needs at any given time is, as we all know a virtual impossibility. Often, the only way that we become aware is via our horse/soma. An active, painful experience will occur, for example a headache, backache, flu or an accident such as one ones Ann and our 13 year old had.

We are in this peculiar configuration in order to cope with an otherwise unmanageable and overwhelming world. We simply cannot consciously contain the endlessness of both the environmental stimuli we are exposed to, nor our internal responses to it and our own unique mindbody chatter. The Rider learns and remembers what is necessary to the present and passes onto the Horse via the Pony Express what they cannot contain. Our Horse's saddlebags produce clues to stresses and pressures we deny and overlook to our detriment. These clues are often only evidenced somatically and generally, painfully. How else would we ever be aware that we might be in danger if our attention was necessarily always focused on a goal? "We" will kick ourselves if we have to like Crystal.

Depending upon how we were looked after as children, by our caregivers, will have a bearing upon how we deal with our inner child/ horse self now. Will we acknowledge the pain signals as meaningful and in need of care? If so, go to bed or get help, or will we ignore them and "soldier on", be brave, because the job is more important? "What doesn't kill us will make us stronger."

Some people will more often whip their own horse and blame it; feeling guilty if they ever admit to a weakness, an attitude most likely learned within their family of origin but filtered into that from the wider community values promulgated by society to ensure we are yoked well to the plough. Others will complain far more vigorously when feeling ill and take to their horse to bed at any sign of adversity. The family of origin care giving behaviors will tell us many interesting stories.

Now within this model, ideally the Stablemaster takes the role of mindfulness of the child's physical, emotional and psychological needs. Over time the child has many thousands of experiences of the parent doing this and is able to develop an inner Stablemaster of their own. When this process, known as Introjection is complete, the inner Stablemaster has been adopted by the developing Rider, integrated into the fabric of the Rider who is then thought of as being able to take responsibility for their Horse for the rest of their life.

This is an ideal because it can never happen perfectly and that is why we have an ongoing internal competition vying for attentions, acting like a Greek Chorus, with the myriad of messages flowing between the horse, introjected stablemaster and rider. Often, whole broadcasts of information are posted; some are read and acknowledged by the rider who is always attempting to be in the saddle directing the flow of life. The Rider is assuming that they are the only one in charge of the whole shooting match; nothing is going to get by them because they are in complete control of every thought, every impulse and every desire. The messages that the rider pays attention to are the ones mainly to do with mapping the path they choose to be on at that time, in that environment, and what tasks need to be carried out.

The introjected Stablemaster might be generating messages about needing supplies for the wellbeing and progress of the self; the rider could be competing with messages generated about wanting to interact with friends, family and social events and work tasks. The messages the horse could be sending might involve going for a good ride and doing the small things like movement, having fun, being spontaneous, sleeping, eating and playing.

There is a never ending parade of headlines to deal with each and every day and they are never exactly the same, they all make a difference and are competing between the systems for top billing!

Becoming Closer to your Own Centre (Centaur) Self-actualization and the Centauring Circle

I will end this chapter with an example that we can use throughout the next few chapters. We have developed an holistic template of assessment, the Centauring Circle, which essentially puts together the ideas we have been discussing up until now with the defence mechanisms evolved within the HR configuration.

Chapter Two will introduce these ideas fully, but for now allow me to introduce you to Mary:

In her mid-thirties Mary had a thriving business that had grown from an acorn of an idea, into an oak tree of work opportunities. She also had a fantastic husband who really loved her, two school age children, three cats, a cockatoo and assorted fish and they all lived a fifty minute one way drive from her workplace. She had a sedentary job of eight hours five days a week; her nights were taken up with cooking, child care and writing work reports with her husband. She felt very tired all the time, sometimes even sick, but never sick enough to take a day off however. Everyone ate breakfast except for Mary, she had a morning liquid diet of five milk based espressos (milk is food, right?), while reading the work mail. Lunch was more coffee and sandwiches. Saturday morning grocery shopping or a three hour drive each way to visit Grandma once a month for the weekend, back for work on Monday morning, dropping the kids off at school; you get the picture.

Looking at this story and the diagram of the Centauring Circle which we will introduce in the next chapter you will see that Mary has some aspects that are glowing with health while others are almost non-existent. She has plenty of family love, work rewards, self-esteem and a lovely home. The one quadrant that missing is the physiological, the horse, which was left in the barn for hours at a time, locked up with talking on phones, on screens and in interviews. That horse was walking not more than ten paces at any given time in a sixteen hour day, it was screaming for release. Not to mention the diet it was subsisting on, the parrot got a much more balanced diet, so did the cats, even the family goldfish did better!

However the messages from the rider and stablemaster were all geared towards looking after others; her inner child's fun consisted of taking the kids to the beach or on a picnic. Mary's horse-self received a hair colour once a month, that she did herself and she felt blessed by the coffee server at the café, because this was the only timeout for her husband and herself from looking after everyone else. I'm sure this is a common story a lot of people share.

Going over the Centauring Circle was for Mary, quite a stunning experience. She found that it was quite hard to believe what she was seeing through this simple, yet holistically integrated analysis. For a woman who was running her own complex and very successful business and who possessed a fabulous intelligence she had to ask some very difficult questions of herself.

Why was she neglecting her horse; why was her diet so poor and her ability to move so restricted? What prevented her from seeing her physical self?

In assessing Mary's psychophysiological lifestyle we must analyse her encrypted messages. These messages are operating at a subliminal or unconscious level which Mary is not consciously aware of. These are the injunctive messages that have almost completely stopped her from active planning for herself.

In doing so we are together teaming up and releasing her horse from its prison.

The next chapter will lead us on an examination of the defence mechanisms. These are the devices expertly used by the Horse and Rider to buck and duck the natural system.

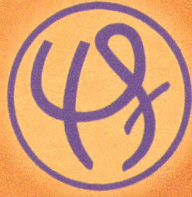

DE-FENCES THAT HINDER AND DE-FENCES THAT HELP
- DE-SIGNING THE JOURNEY TO THE CENTAUR -

'History, like repression, is never over, just because it's in the past.'

Sara Beaumont-Connop

In Chapter 1 we asked why we were in the particular configuration HR comes in and we arrived at some remarkable conclusions, not the least was the Horse and Rider (HR) saddlebag system. This system allows us to survive in the world, to work through what the world throws at us while making the best decisions we can out of what we perceive and feel. This system has many built in ways of coping, each belonging to the duality of the HR as they have their own interacting defensive systems. We all need these internal defensive capabilities to deal with the otherwise overwhelming life stimuli that are encountered and responded to every day. We could see these as life's hurdles that the HR have defenses to engage, a lot like your own personal steeple chase.

We are in this particular configuration as it is our only method of coping, however we cannot simply stuff the saddlebags full forever without paying a fairly fatal penalty and hence we have our psychophysiological gifts for coping (Defences) which give us survival techniques that we are quite often unaware of.

One of the best defensive systems and probably the most ignored consciously, whenever

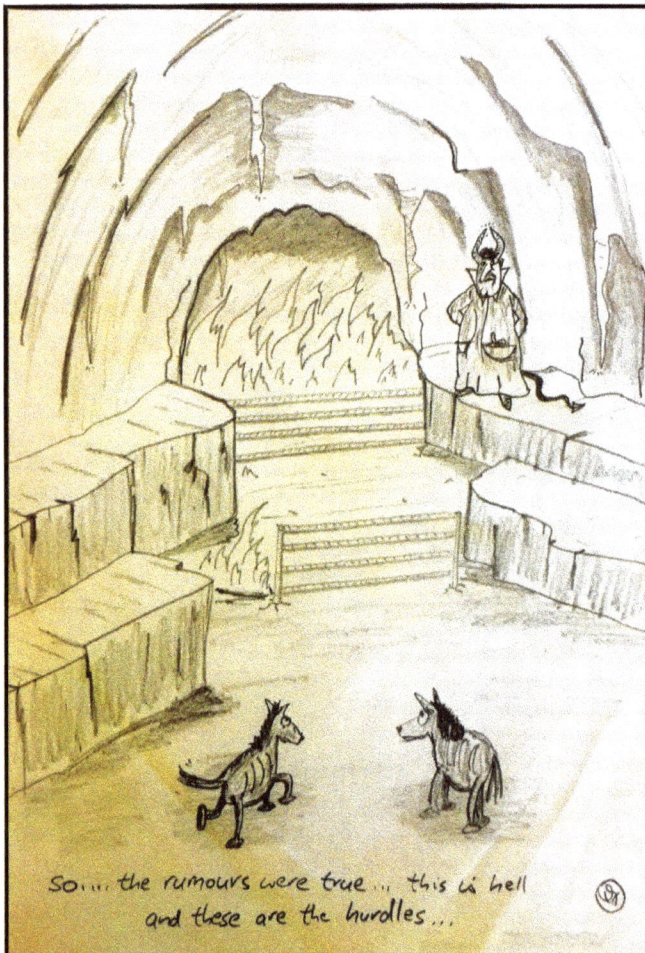

So... the rumours were true ... this is hell and these are the hurdles...

possible, is the physical manifestation of pain. Our Horse has a multitude of systems at its disposal to characterise adversity reactions. These defenses are symbolised in a hierarchical order just as the defenses of the mind (Rider) are, and react to the level of the adversary being engaged.

We have been using these since we were born, for example the startle response when a sudden noise happens or crying with colic or hunger, which demand engagement and interpretation in order to produce resolution! Some defenses have become more elaborate, more elusive and difficult for the conscious mind to understand and respond to. These may present as a physical manifestation when their etiology is psychological stress. These can include things like the development of a rash, neck pains or sudden craving for foods (outside of pregnancy).

We have developed these physical defenses along with psychological defenses in tandem and over our childhood, adolescence and adulthood they evolved as we were presented with more hurdles to jump, more problems to solve and more skills to develop.

Why do we need physical defenses, why can't we just solve every issue with our minds? The simplest answer to this in my opinion is that our ingenious holistic nature allows us three different threads of awareness:

The Three Natures

Looking at the psychophysiological development of a person we find the Horse and Rider configuration. I would like to call this evolution of our selves the Centaur for simplicity and within this Centaur lie the potential three natures.

The **first nature** is the awareness and potential personality that the child is born with and it emanates from our mind. This growing awareness develops from understanding "part objects", like the difference, for instance, between our arm and our mother's breast. Many of you will have seen something like surprise and wonder passing over an infant's face as it sees its own arm moving over its head as it lies on its back. This "surprise" occurs because the infant, at this age, does not have awareness yet of its own extension in space and so, sees the arm as an object separate from itself! This is the nature which makes sense out of the environment, both internal and external.

The **second nature** is concerned with the developing infant gaining control and mastery over their own bodily functions, such as lifting their heads, sitting up, crawling, climbing, walking, running and so on, leading to a full mastery of the physical self. This nature is concerned with control and mastery over the environment. These two natures are on parallel bands throughout a person's lifetime.

The **third nature** is also threaded through developmental lines and is awareness which only emanates from the harmonious combination of the first two natures. This is transmuted into a motivational creativity allowing the person to be truly in the moment in a joyous and uplifted way, managing tasks and adversity masterfully. Some people quantify it as spirituality, some call it creativity, Maslow called it actualisation and it has been described as the Kung Fu of any activity by the ancient Chinese. This third nature produces our individual belief systems and as it generates we can get elevated and motivated and the harmonic of the three natures produces our higher self, the Centaur. A good example of a person who achieved this is Nelson Mandela, his life's work constantly gave him opportunities to use his mind and body to centaur himself and achieve higher goals even under extreme deprivation and hardships. Centauring, even in the prison, he was able to harmoniously produce energy sufficient to overcome his hardships and as he said: "Tension is the enemy of serenity, and exercise dissipates tension".

I believe that we all have a unique individual perspective and awareness of something not being quite right within our physical being; we don't feel centaured. You have to agree that this is a part of yourself (the physical) that you have lived with all your life! Who else has felt tired for you, hungry for you, pain for you!? Only your mother, linked through the special attachment relationship developed in the first years of your life, generated what is known as a primary maternal preoccupation with you. This psychophysiological bond was made with you only to help you to create your own internal psychophysiological bond. Then its handed on to you, an intergenerational pattern yes, but everything about your centaur is truly your own; fingerprints, toe prints, eye retinal patterns, thoughts and feelings, no one else will ever be you.

So, not feeling centaured within ourselves is the strongest clue that there is something wrong and careful examination of our defenses will lead to the discovery of what it is.

The unusual life that we experience as the HR brings with it duality of feelings. Horse physicality and Rider metaphysicality encapsulates an interdimensional dilemma that can only be engaged holistically.

It is the wisdom of the experience that comes of living within the individual HR duality that gives us this opportunity for holistic growth. We do know and feel when something is wrong with us, even if we don't know exactly what that is.

I believe that this faith that we can have in our own ability to know ourselves is our greatest strength in developing coping strategies when it comes to adversity and living our lives holistically. We will follow no path but our own anyway!

You can lead a horse to water but you can't make it drink!

Physical Defences: Acknowledging and Integrating the Horse

We are considering another fundamental point of difference in HR, that of the ontological being of the Horse and its defence mechanisms. These defenses develop in a linked and parallel process to those of the Riders, the psychological defence mechanisms.

We cannot have psychological defence actions or reactions without there ever being a physical paralleling mirror, nor can we experience a physical defence engaging without having a psychological parallel. We are HR and we live in a world of duality even though all of us are frequently operating as though we live only in the world of the Rider! We are in a state of denial regarding our second nature, the world of our Horse, our physicality, and yet we are constantly receiving input from it as a psychophysiological being. So how are we actually coping with this?

Please refer to diagram opposite: Developmental Evolution of HR Defences.

The diagrammatic representation of our defence mechanisms has the infants earliest responses shown at the centre left. The startle response, crying, gurgling and smiling naturally progress through attachment to a loving caregiver and we evolve in a parallel development towards the right of the diagram with the Rider above and the Horse below.

Throughout the childhood, adolescence and early adulthood our defence maturity hopefully develops; hopefully, because without caring and appropriate caregivers we do not follow a normal course of development, we cannot do so by ourselves.

Our defence mechanisms are developmental. We have evolved over millennia and quite

THE RIDER'S DIMENSION — REALM OF THE MIND — PSYCHOLOGICAL	ENVIRONMENTAL PRESSURES IMPACTING RIDER PARALLEL HORSE IN H&R DUALITY	Developmental Evolution of Psychophysiological Defence Mechanisms	FAMILY NEEDS — SOCIAL GROUP PRESSURE — FRIENDS, PEERS EMPLOYMENT	ACCEPTANCE OF AGEING AND SOCIETIES RESPONSE — RETIREMENT CHALLENGES
	5. 6. 7. 8. 9. 10.	15. 20. 30	40. 50. 60	70. 80. 90+
Enjoyment and contentment of closeness and feeding. Reflection of smiling faces	Developing strong and intense friendships: identification; magical thinking; guilt; repression; splitting of self; regression to earlier stage; denial, blame; imaginary friends; acting out	Dissociation; intellectualisation Rationalisation, acceptance; Humour; identification Gratitude; courage, respect Sublimation suppression	Continuation of all of the positive, mature defences when centauring and all of the less mature, regressive defences when unable to.	Continuation
BIRTH BRINGS PRIMARY DEFENCES ONLY				

THE HORSE'S DIMENSION — SPHERE OF THE BODY — PHYSICAL	ENVIRONMENTAL PRESSURES IMPACTING HORSE PARALLEL RIDER IN H&R DUALITY	ENVIRONMENT EXTERNAL REALITY PHYSICAL LIVING COSTS TO ORGANISM	AGE RELATED HEALTH ISSUES AND CHANGES TO THE PHYSICAL ABILITIES AND CAPACITIES OF THE YOUNGER HORSE	ADAPTATION TO CHANGE
Crying out loud Startle response	Crying; conversion disorders like sore tummy, headaches, feeling sick and unwell; anxiety, sleeplessness, nightmares and night terrors	Conversion of kinetic anxiety into focused thought and constructive action through the use of conscious movement and exercise of the body attuned to the moment.	Continuation of all of the positive when centauring and all of the negative when unable to	Continuation
Awareness of anxiety and the physical expression of pain and discomfit.				

possibly, for instance, we needed denial and minimisation as survival tools while hunting. Our focus on the prey of utmost importance, denial and minimisation operating in the background to filter out distractions which would otherwise wreck our chances of success and raise the likelihood of not surviving.

As we have socialised in greater and greater intensity our complexity has evolved our defences by necessity. These mechanisms are our keys to survival as we have already seen in chapter one. We are in this configuration in order to manage being here but we pay a cost for it: our saddlebags can contain the pain but not forever, we will examine more closely later in the book just how these bags are able to be engaged and released, but for the rest of this chapter we are going to look at some of the principle de-fences we have de-signed in order to see just how we manage in our world and we will illustrate them using cases which have had every identifiable feature removed but which are all remarkably true. In each example note the beauty of the parallel messaging system operating within the HR duality.

Body discomfort and pain are the first line of the Horses defence as we are all aware! We are unavoidably physically hardwired through the brain stem and throughout every cell of our body to feel and react to pain. A baby will cry out immediately in pain as children exhibit pain as a whole body experience more freely than adults. The meaning of pain has been studied more than virtually anything else given how easily it attracts our attention! Obviously accidents are environmental activators of pain and are as such considered separately, but there are many more reasons for pain and physical discomfort to manifest itself.

Everyone has a different reaction and threshold for pain and it is always contingent on the antecedents, whether or not they are psychological or physical as to their meaning. We are however primarily working with ordinary health issues and learning to harness the potential positive messages that our physical defenses are indicating to us, as a preventative response and life enhancing opportunity.

Anxiety for instance, is a universal experience to fear of pain or discomfit, and can be seen in the multitude physical dimensions such as breathing difficulties, inability to move, sweating, dizziness, rashes and racing heart for instance.

We have seen that our body can act as a great amphitheatre for the storage and retrieval of historical pains and traumatic physical and psychological events. These are all recorded with Shakespearian accuracy somewhere in the saddlebags. If John broke his collarbone twice when he was a teenager and it healed even though he could not see it, the fact of it breaking painfully and the ensuing traumatic experience of recovery was classified in his physical library under the history section. Now, when he calls on his shoulder 30 years later to act in physical play the event on record does make itself known as part of his physical character. It enacts the trauma as weakness and sometimes as pain and an inability to function in the way John is attempting to operate. This unconsciously retrieved information is acted out in John's life by impeding his wishes to physically move and operate in ways he desires. It is limiting John even though there is no longer any physical damage nor any physical impediment; there is recorded however, within the classified section, the possibility of damage and that is the anchor which needs attention. The dramas that our various body pains like an aching back, severe neck pain, migraine headaches, twisting and griping stomach aches and any manner of physical torment that we experience, can all emanate from our present or our past. Our feedback system relies on our focus and analysis in order to understand these messages, as the Rider, through these unconscious connections to the Horse, exists partially outside of the ordinary concept of time! History, in these cases always repeats!

We will briefly run through most of the common defence mechanisms illustrating them with stories demonstrating their operations. At the end of this section we will align them within the Centauring Circle and see the incredible symmetry HR have for potential holistic health.

Denial

One of the most primary, yet most often utilised of our defenses is denial. Children develop the defence of denial at an extraordinarily early age and are prepared to use it at any time to the frequent disbelief of their parents, caregivers or teachers.

The denial of pain or even of physical events can be characterised in a myriad of ways: an actress who was overweight was interviewed about her weight gain and why she did not appear to notice a 30kg increase. She replied that when she ate, often in front of the television set, she wore elastic waisted baggy pants, so the pants stretched without discomfort and she could continue watching TV and not need to acknowledge and therefore not see the reality she was creating even though it was as an attempt from one part of herself to signal distress to another part of herself.

We are primarily concerned with stress and trauma related suffering that can be alleviated with a concerted HR holistic approach. It has been shown over and over again that the improvement of any living things internal or external environment does promote a growth towards the positive. For example, thirty five years ago psychopaedic wards existed. These wards were not for mainstream psychiatric patients, they were designed for people born with special needs such as intellectual and physical disabilities combined. One such ward existed for children who were extremely disabled and it had a very high death rate. I was invited to participate in a special program that the director had devised. It was simply called the Holding Program. Every day some volunteers would go into the ward and pick up a child that had been assigned to them. For several hours we would hold the child, rock them, talk to them, stroke their hair, doing everything a mother would do with her infant. By the end of 6 months the death rate dramatically dropped in that ward, all the children were thriving, they were responding to their environment, moving and articulating towards their caregivers, they were not lying silently in purgatory anymore.

When we consider the developmentally related defence mechanisms in the above diagram in the light of Bowlby's attachment theory as shown in chapter 1 we can see how such a basic change might bring about such a remarkable difference in these children's lives and yet it was seemingly too difficult to do for many years.

Denial is one of the first defenses we use in conscious life as children yet it remains one of the most utilized defenses in the unexamined lives we lead as adults. It is the primary defence used by perpetrators in domestic violence settings and is closely followed by blaming others and minimization; more about these follows later.

A Rash Story

An interesting and fascinating feature of our saddlebags is their storage capacity and what we carry unknowingly from the past that nevertheless physically manifests in our present without our awareness of the meaning of it and where it comes from. There was a woman who went to see her doctor every autumn for a recurring skin rash. Strangely, it only occurred for one month of autumn, but it always manifested horrendously for the month and drove her crazy with the itching. No cream seemed to work on it, no allergy medicine either and the doctor in desperation referred her to a skin specialist to no avail. The woman was by now getting desperate herself and was referred to a psychotherapist who worked next door to the skin specialist. After taking a thorough assessment and during the therapy she began to have a dream about an orchard where she had worked as a teenager picking apples. As the woman progressed in her therapy, she retrieved memories of being attacked in the orchard by a male worker who sexually assaulted her. She cried as she remembered how the hard ground and dead leaves and twigs had scrapped and scratched her back, exactly where the rash materialized each autumn. After her conscious mind had the cathartic release from the pain of the traumatic memory, the woman no longer needed to physically manifest the rash as a reminder and angry demand for her trauma to be heard and acted on and so the rash disappeared.

The events of the assault were at the time of their occurrence too overwhelming for the young woman to relate to anyone; she was able through the Rider's defenses to put them out of her conscious memory eventually. The Horse however was unable to completely contain the abusive information and through its actions her body told a story of anger and rash. This story needed to be understood correctly and was repeated for some years until it was heard.

The parallel systems of the HR duality communicate without pause and continue to search for harmony when there is none.

Accidents Harming Self

Remember our friend Crystal and her injured ankle? Upon reciting to me what was occurring at her work place, she realized she had uttered the words "I feel like I don't have a leg to stand on" while attempting to deal with the problems confronting her, especially with the work colleague and his stalking behaviour. It is ironic that the accident that Crystal suffered meant she was unable to go to work for some time giving her respite from her fears. Crystal's anxiety had been translated into a physical action, which while harmful to her, meant that she avoided a potentially dangerous environment. Nevertheless it had translated into a masochistic wounding for her that obviously was a painful and unhealthy hobbling.

Immune System Problems, Recurrent Flu, Illnesses

Every time Bob and Wendy took a week off from their joint business, they both got the flu, not a major flu, but the kind that starts with a headache, then a bit of a sore throat followed by sneezing and tiredness. It kept them at home lying around feeling 'run down', they had both felt fine at work, toiling away sixteen hours a day, it just seemed to hit them whenever they tried to stop and relax. Very much like a toxin that built up over time, being stored in the lymph nodes, released as they gave their physical selves an opportunity to breathe out, after holding that breath, living on adrenaline to get their work done. It was as if their Horse was biting them back after its captivity.

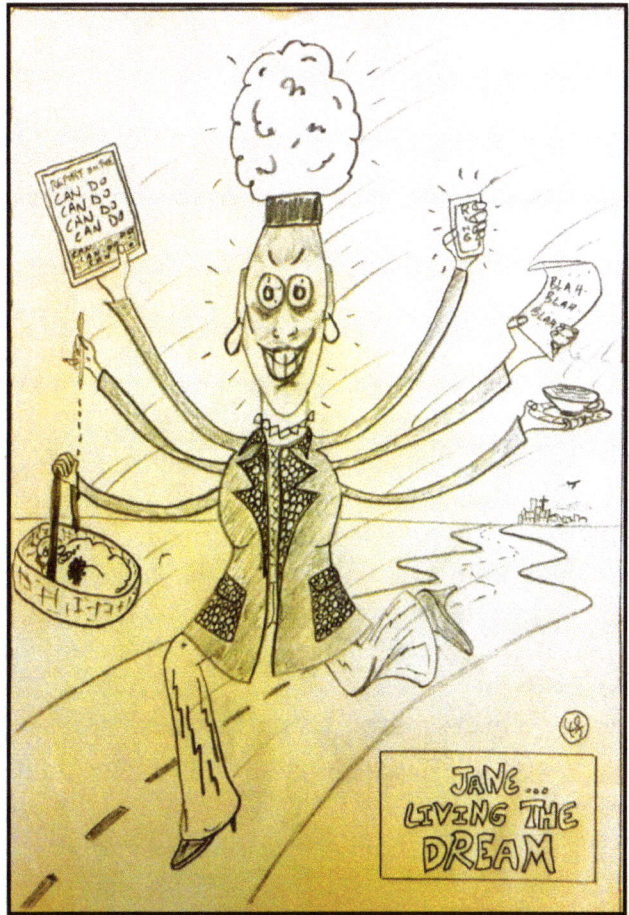

JANE... LIVING THE DREAM

Crying, Feelings of Depression, and Inability to carry out Tasks

Jane got to the end of her working day, slumped in the uncomfortable office chair. She scrolled down the pages of email messages and glanced at the lists of reports due. A wave of tiredness washed over, pricking her eyes with tears, "I can't do it!" A small voice wailed in her mind, "it's just too much!" At five thirty on the way home Jane stopped at the corner store, she'd had a sandwich for lunch and nothing else all day. Five bags of assorted sweets later, Jane continued her drive home to make the family dinner, tears running down her cheeks, chewing wine-gums and pineapple lumps in quick succession, it began to get very dark those last few miles as she drove home. She awoke the next morning to the uncomfortable reality of yet another yeast infection to deal with, the final straw, the moment of crisis, the horse had spoken! Jane rang a midwife friend who sent her a book on the connection between sugar addition and yeast infections along with some holistic diet alternatives. Desperate to be well, Jane followed the books recommendations. The infections cleared up, she began to lose weight, feel better and remember how good jogging made her feel in the past. The first steps were baby ones, starting from crawl, it hurt, she stumbled, but got up; her mantra began "just do 10 minutes and see how you feel", "just a little further you can do it!" The weeks went by and Jane got up in the mornings and ran into the sun rise, the beginning of a new way.

Failure to Thrive, or Doing the Same Thing over and over and Expecting a Different Outcome

Imagine this every day you wake up a different person, not because you planned this the day before but because imperceptibly our physicality changes, not because you wanted it to but it is our second nature, the nature of the Horse. Without doing anything skin cells fell off, cells divided, hair grew; a metamorphosis of you was taking place. We cannot go back on this journey, we can only go forward; again, in the natural order of the universe, energy moves changes and becomes.

The fact, that however much we may like to see, a separateness from our physicality, we cannot as we are manifesting as a duality, HR is configured ontologically in this way. We can be potentially centaured in it. We walk and talk our way into it every day!

If we can decipher the physical messages our horse is sending us, these can give us information to help deal with life in a more holistic way. It is true that these are the one signals we medicate the most to shut down! These messages, however carry valuable insight into what our individual repertoire of ailments are and how we are currently coping with adversities. Understanding that physicality is not a choice, rather it is a given; that we cannot change horses in mid-stream, nor should we look our gift horse in the mouth. We may have an internal library however it does come with an external exchange system.

Preventative holistic health provides opportunities to ride or divide off tensions (cathartically) that are overwhelming the centaur preventing movement and causing disparity between the physical and the psychological, the HR. Unfortunately we often wait for a physical crisis leading to a psychological crisis before attending to our centaur. I call these Kinetic negative energies, which are interpreted by the HR by using defence mechanisms both physical and psychological stored in our library of thought and movement.

Even our posture denotes the carriage of our despair or joy; what's in our saddlebags both past and present and as we shall see later, it is an excellent evaluative tool.

Compartmentalisation is a specific defence which boxes away many of the things causing us anxiety, like the old story of Pandora's Box. When we use it to neutralise our physical defence systems, we immobilise them with the numbing effects of, for instance: medication, food, alcohol, drugs, or screens and in doing so, our second nature, the Horse, is disconnected and becomes split off from what we will call the "Mind's eye". At this point even a mirror is unable to facilitate an integrative equation of the duality of HR, so all that is seen in the reflection of the mirror is the head! We choose one rather than both.

As it is in all universal truths, so too it is here, that everything is made up of positive and negative energies and we are no different in this regard. A dichotomous arrangement of yes verses no, good verses bad, sit down verses stand up, being still verses movement, silence verses noise, to do something or to do nothing confronts us eternally.

The continuous struggle with what appears to be presented to us as a choice between these two paths has lead me to write this book about how to put something into action instead of choosing either the path of reaction or the path of inaction.

Make the journey with the third path which develops out of the first two and discover a constant compass which we can use in response to any adversities faced.

Centauring Circle: The Psychophysiological Defence Shield

At the end of chapter 1 we introduced the term "Centauring Circle" along with Mary's story. It's now time to introduce the CC as we continue our exploration of the psychophysiological defenses.

In this first introduction to the CC *(See diagram on following page)* you will see a wheel of behaviours and feelings potentially expressed when interacting with life. We are describing these as our defenses and some of these defensive strategies are better than others. For example, imagine being a warrior of old carrying the CC as a shield for protection, the shield is an amalgamation of wood and iron; if you hold it up in some positions it operates in a more powerful way when dealing with adversity than in other positions. Which position would you want to operate most in, when faced with lives challenges?

A hierarchy of maturity ranks the CC ability in making better quality defenses, the ones that are more effect and integrative than the other less evolved ones. These systems work in a spiraling formation, like the shield, sometimes the wooden aspects of the shield are sufficient, such as denying the fact you were 10 mins late for work, however this would not be sufficient to deal with being 2 hours late for work! Using the lesser effective ways of coping with hurdles can mean that the self is rendered into a splintered state as wood cannot stand up to some serious situations, thus rendering the person more anxious than before and possibly more likely to act out in ways that lead to destructive behaviours towards themselves and others.

"Shields Up"

This inbuilt shield interacts with our reality all the time with messages from the outside being relayed to the HR, they produce our conscious thoughts and feelings from the underlying stream of information flowing within both Horse and Rider dimensions which are constantly interacting with the inner and outer world. Simultaneously the shield comes into play effecting our decisions on how to behave, essentially what to say or do.

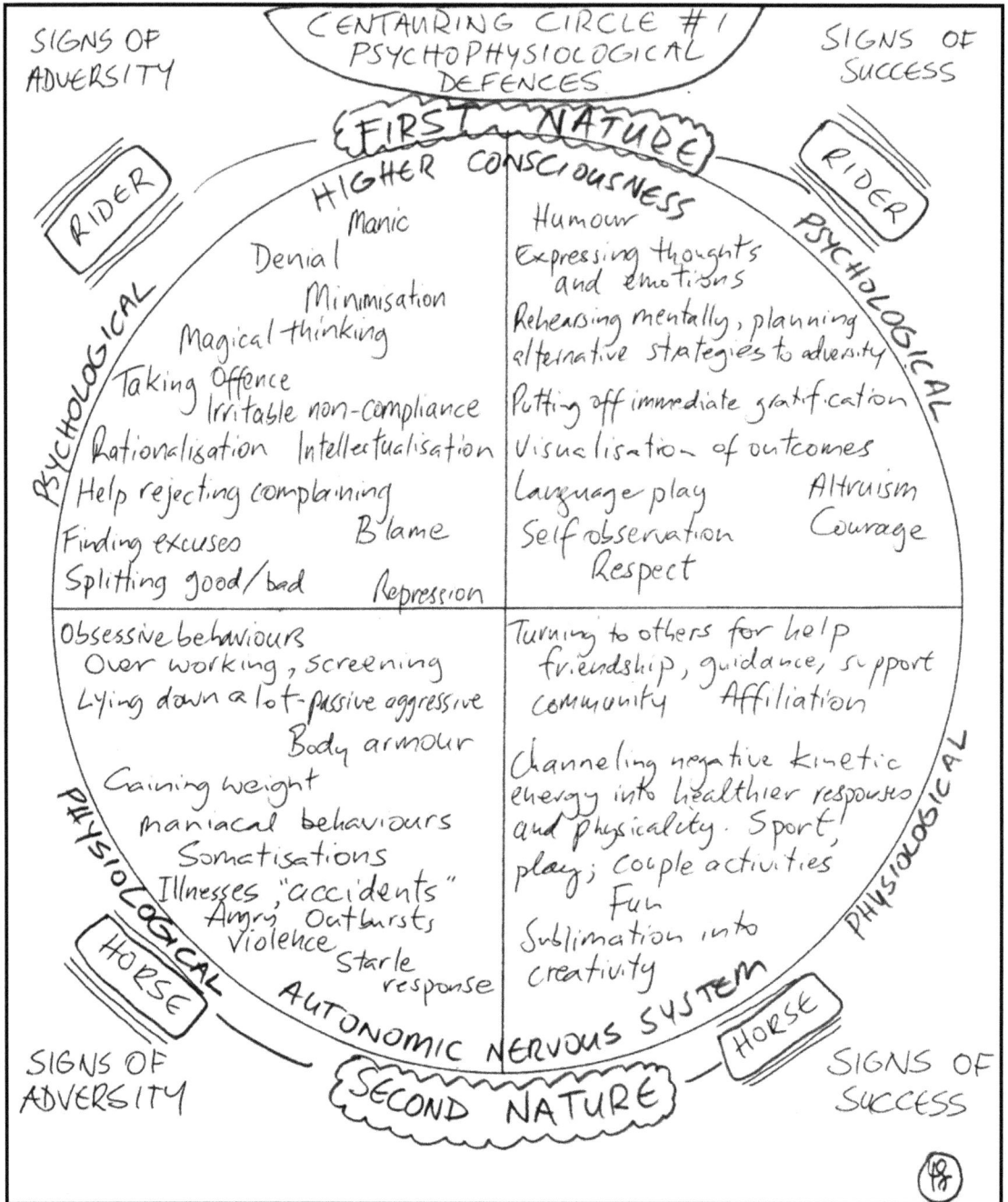

CENTAURING CIRCLE #1
PSYCHOPHYSIOLOGICAL
DEFENCES

SIGNS OF ADVERSITY

SIGNS OF SUCCESS

FIRST NATURE

HIGHER CONSCIOUSNESS

RIDER — PSYCHOLOGICAL

Left upper (Signs of Adversity — Psychological):
Manic
Denial
Minimisation
Magical thinking
Taking Offence
Irritable non-compliance
Rationalisation Intellectualisation
Help rejecting complaining
Finding excuses   Blame
Splitting good/bad   Repression

Right upper (Signs of Success — Psychological):
Humour
Expressing thoughts and emotions
Rehearsing mentally, planning alternative strategies to adversity
Putting off immediate gratification
Visualisation of outcomes
Language play   Altruism
Self observation   Courage
Respect

Left lower (Signs of Adversity — Physiological):
Obsessive behaviours
Over working, screening
Lying down a lot-passive aggressive
Body armour
Gaining weight
maniacal behaviours
Somatisations
Illnesses "accidents"
Angry Outbursts
Violence
Startle response

Right lower (Signs of Success — Physiological):
Turning to others for help friendship, guidance, support
community   Affiliation
Channeling negative kinetic energy into healthier responses and physicality. Sport, play; couple activities
Fun
Sublimation into creativity

AUTONOMIC NERVOUS SYSTEM

HORSE — PHYSIOLOGICAL

SECOND NATURE

SIGNS OF ADVERSITY

SIGNS OF SUCCESS

This Defensive Shield is Divided up into Four Quadrants

The left side of the shield are the basic defenses that we have used all of our lives at some point to deal with realities issues, I have divided this half of the shield into 2 quadrants, number one quadrant at the top of the shield is made up of the riders defensive thoughts and feelings which may or may not be expressed fully consciously or verbally; the bottom quadrant is the horse's arena containing the active behaviours that are physical manifestations of defensive positions we adopt.

Examples of these Defences are:

Denying the issue (denial): Roy had been coming home to cheese and sherry every day after work for eighteen months. He just wanted complete calm, he did not want to see or hear the children or to talk, period! To polite enquiry, work was fine, everything was fine! Roy looked like a volcano about to erupt, calmly sipping sherry, cutting off slices of cheddar and swooshing the newspaper, from page to page. Denying anything was wrong and oozing from every pore, like lava, before 'the Big One!

Taking Offence: Two women, friends for years, were talking about their lifestyles. The first woman was following a paleo diet and exercising regularly, the other woman was not. During the course of the conversation the second woman became very agitated and suddenly accusing the first woman of telling her she was fat and lazy! The first woman was stunned, taken aback and mystified as she put down the phone after her friend had hung up on her. She had not mentioned anything about her friend's behaviour in any way.

Giving long explanations that really mean nothing is going to change (rationalizing) "On yer Bike": Recently and at his wife's request, Ross bought a bike as all their friends had bikes. They used them nearly every day and exhorted Ross and his wife to ride with them. Ross had ridden a great deal in his twenties, as he painstakingly explained to the friends and his wife. His car had been stolen, he had no insurance and no money for a new car. A friend lent him a ten speed bike, he rode that bike, rain, hail, sun or sleet, every day for years. It was grueling but Ross had ridden his iron steed up hell hill and back! He could tell that tale for hours, while the new bike stayed safe in the garage!

Making the issue smaller (minimization) "The expanding trousers" A wife was anxiously evaluating her husband's seemingly expanding waistline, her husband was disputing her claims at every turn. Each time she started to talk about his possibly expanding girth, he would get a pair of trousers out of his wardrobe, hold them up and triumphantly announce that these pants were "getting too big for him, his waist was really shrinking". This miracle of nature was occurring without any lifestyle changes at all!

Help Rejecting Complaining or "No thank you, this hurts!"

For a long time Abby sat languishing on the cliffs of despair, feeling tired and sluggish. "I'm only 35 years old she cried; I should be fine!" Teetering on the edge, Abby would painstakingly list all of her responsibilities: her job, her children, her pets, her garden and just for good measure she would throw in the kitchen sink!

"Oh yes"! She wept, swaying sideways. "It's all there!" Hours of sitting at work, children with school issues, trouble with her sister, a bad diet and still building a new home! On and on she droned out the issues. Carefully grasping her husband's ear as he came up to the surface of his ocean for air. She wailed and moaned, a siren close to the rocks of calamity. Any lifeline thrown, ignored! Abby would rather sink down under the waves of sea of her familiar adversity, drowning in rhetoric, she had control!

Blaming Other People or Situations (Avoidance)

The situation most blamed for lack of change is the lack of time, usually due to work hours combined with not enough help with home based responsibilities. Here's an example of a typical conversation opener a lot of personal trainers get when discussing regular exercise routines:

"I'm so busy" Joan sighed, "I can never get the time to go to the gym, there is always a job to do, then I'm too tired and John is no help, he likes to go out to rugby practice twice a week. Then there is Friday night drinks with friends and trying to get baby sitters, Saturday morning shopping, cleaning the house. I want to lose weight and feel better; I get so many tension headaches, but you can see, it's really not my fault, there is no time and no one to help at home!

These are simple examples of the Rider using ineffective but defensive styles against adversity. When we are tired, overwrought and stressed they are easy to use but often lead to poor outcomes for ourselves as individuals and within our couple and familial relationships.

As we can see opposite, in the Adversity Graph, these are the long term results of using poor strategies and are indicative of an individual who really needs help.

The second quadrant of the shield on the lower left belongs to the realm of the Horse's physicality. These behaviours are usually obvious to the outside observer as they are the visibly acted out aspects which correspond to the Rider's less than brilliant choices under stress.

Some of these actions we very evident in Crystal's story at the beginning of the book, can you identify any of them?

Some other examples are:

Avoidant Defences

Obsessive behaviours such as overworking, excessive shopping, spending too much time and money on internet gaming, binge drinking and eating. Often when we feel much stressed, or

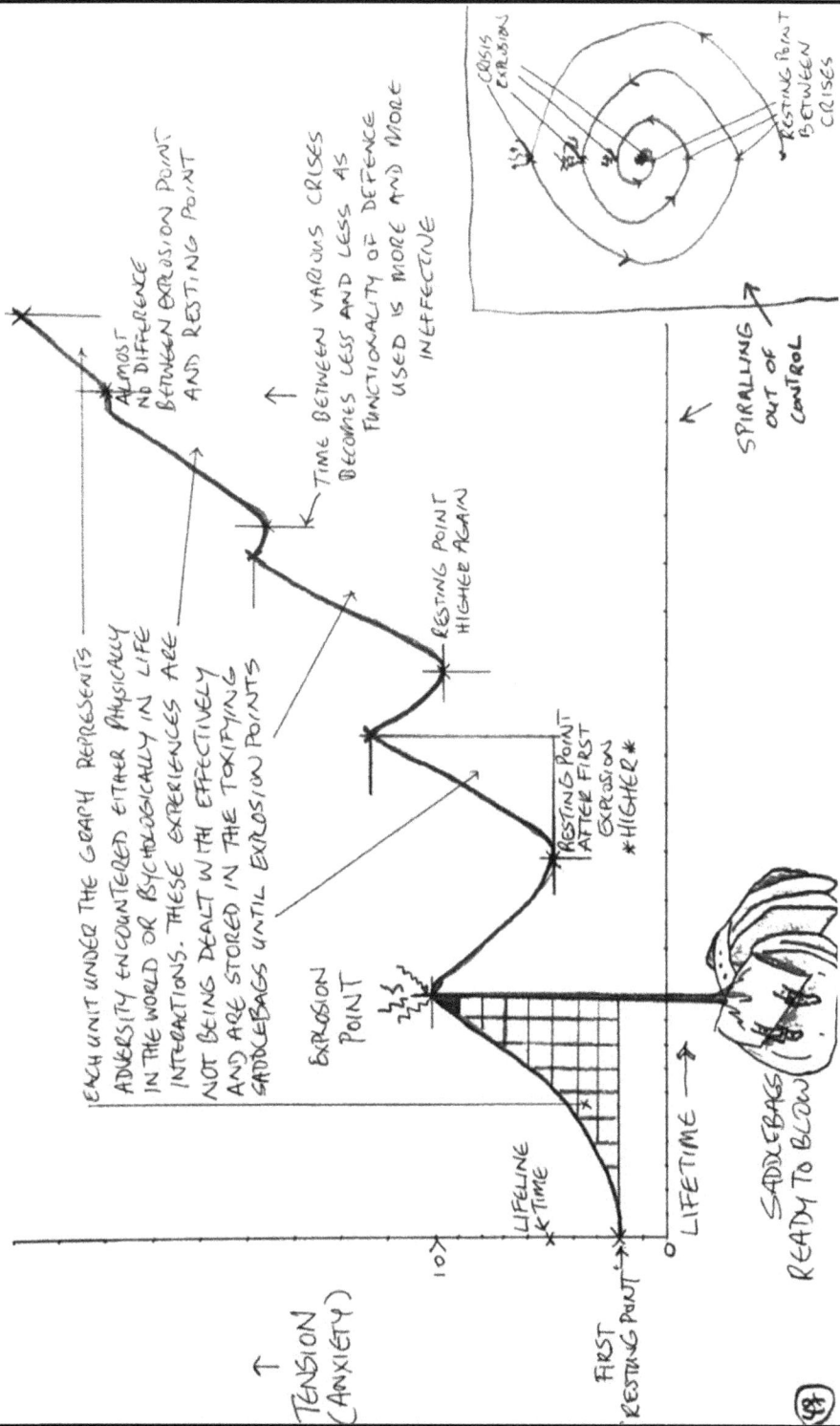

"GRAPH OF DISASTERS WITH ADVERSITY" or DEFENCE MECHANISMS GONE WRONG
(SEE TEXT)

TENSION (ANXIETY)

EACH UNIT UNDER THE GRAPH REPRESENTS ADVERSITY ENCOUNTERED EITHER PHYSICALLY IN THE WORLD OR PSYCHOLOGICALLY IN LIFE INTERACTIONS. THESE EXPERIENCES ARE NOT BEING DEALT WITH EFFECTIVELY AND ARE STORED IN THE TOXIFYING SADDLEBAGS UNTIL EXPLOSION POINTS

ALMOST NO DIFFERENCE BETWEEN EXPLOSION POINT AND RESTING POINT

TIME BETWEEN VARIOUS CRISES BECOMES LESS AND LESS AS FUNCTIONALITY OF DEFENCE USED IS MORE AND MORE INEFFECTIVE

RESTING POINT HIGHER AGAIN

RESTING POINT AFTER FIRST EXPLOSION *HIGHER*

EXPLOSION POINT

LIFELINE ∝ TIME

10

LIFETIME →

FIRST RESTING POINT

0

SADDLEBAGS READY TO BLOW

CRISIS EXPLOSION

RESTING POINT BETWEEN CRISES

SPIRALLING OUT OF CONTROL

experience an emptiness or deficit within our self, these emotions can be relayed to the physical self. The corresponding active message back, Horse to Rider, involve what we sometimes call "acting out". These behaviours are frequently used to "block out" other, real but unwanted thoughts and real world pressures. They serve us in the short term to seem to ourselves, and others, to be OK however, they can never serve us in a medium or long term measure as effective because they are at best deceptive means to avoid something unavoidable.

A Modern Day Fairy Story

Back in the day, computers in the Antipodes were relatively new, Apple was only beginning to mean an inorganic item! Jack's mother had just purchased a home computer, she saw it as an upmarket typewriter. Jack was eleven and fascinated with this new technology. The hours Jack spent pouring over this Pandora's Box, at night when his mother thought him asleep were innumerable. Jack's parents had separated and Jack was worried throughout his days about what would happen because of this. He had been losing sleep at night as well, but since the computer arrived everything had changed. Every morning Jack awoke to view his screen, every day he spent dreaming in algorithmic space and in the evening he had computing designs to try out as he ate his dinner alone in his room with the computer. The school holidays came, Jack was twelve; he went to his mother's workplace, a library within a large city council. Jack's mother shelved books whilst Jack was given her password to use her work computer. Jack laughed to himself about the encrypted games he and the computer could play; games most adults did not know, a language that they had not yet learnt. This machine spoke especially to Jack so he did not need friends or sport or hobbies, he had this secret world to explore and hide in, to run to when he was angry or scared or lonely, a place that only a few like him could get to. Jack tested himself that day in the library; he entered the maze at the centre of his mother's computer and left a tiny graffiti right in its heart: a magic bean that could grow silently for several years unheeded and unnoticed. A plant that when harvested could supply Jack with access to all the giant's money.

Jack was fourteen when the fraud squad audited the library's computer on a tip off and found the bean stalk and his dumbfounded mother was led away for questioning.

All of the defenses depend upon the degree of anxiety stimulated by the perceived reality situation that the individual feels they are dealing with. Some of them are conscious, some preconscious and others unconscious. Another example of active defensive behaviour can be noted as coping.

Coping Mechanisms

Putting on Body Armour: this can occur if an outside reality situation becomes dangerous to the Rider and the Horse. The whole system goes into major psychophysiological defensive reaction. For example, a small boy is bullied at school, he is too weak to fight the bigger boys off. At 13 years old he finds the gym and begins to work out with weights. The more he works out, the more muscle he develops and the more the other boys leave him alone. Realising the quality of defence this armour gives him, he continues to build his physic at the gym which in turn leads him into competitive body building.

Somatic Storage of Trauma

Putting on weight can be a reaction to grief, depression or physical trauma of any kind, especially abuse. We may not consciously remember what started or triggered the journey to the physical defence we have set up as this is usually locked in the classified section of our library and forgotten or repressed, however we play it out by our actions and our physiology.

Even our posture can manifest as an active indicator of how the HR is feeling. When we are tired, we often slump forward, caving at the chest or we have tight stiff neck muscles from sitting at a screen focusing. We very often seem to forget to stop long enough to take a breath and stretch our cramped up bodies!

The Fantasy world that screens enable us to inhabit, disengages linear time psychologically. Screens, particularly the higher resolution varieties have successfully joined the defence of compartmentalisation of our thought processing. This process enables us to inhabit a cube of space-time outside of normal life and is seen as a dissociative state. This state of being is acting as an insulation which becomes protective against negative thoughts, feelings and realities internally as well as putting on blinkers to any external realities that we want to block out at that time.

Having Accidents and other Extreme Messages from H to R

Crystal, at the beginning of our story, was a good example of not having a "leg to stand on" when she damaged her ankle accidentally. There are a million examples to choose from in illustrating this, even as Freud himself said: "there are no such things as accidents". We do disagree with this, however he was on to something particularly striking. Often when overburdened, the Horse will crash and this is seen as accidental. Whenever we look at the burdens, however, quite often it is remarkable that some sort of "accident" hasn't already occurred. We have all heard of the phrase: "an accident just waiting to happen" unfortunately.

If we are using a defence pattern from the poorer side of the Centauring Circle for a long enough period of time, we are going to encounter a crisis point. These crisis points occur either whenever the saddlebags are at their breaking point, stuffed full of unresolved issues and conflicts, or, when we are interacting with real adversity and choosing poor behaviours. Please refer to the Adversity Graph.

Whenever one of these circumstances is occurring some sort of "accident" will happen, usually accompanied by phrases like: "I didn't mean it"; "I didn't think it could be so bad"," It was only a small push, they fell over the stool there", etc.

Angry outbursts are another example of the above and will always occur as the gradient of the Adversity Graph steepens and approaches crisis point.

Illnesses, for example developing an ulcer and getting the flu frequently are also examples of messages from Horse to Rider.

The Inconvenient Tooth

Mr Ed had been having trouble with his back molar tooth for some time, he had attended to it several years ago by having a root canal procedure done, however, it had still been hurting when he ate. During his busy schedule, he felt a sore in his mouth, on the same side as the problem tooth, an ulcer, he concluded, even though he did not really get ulcers and he did not check to see if it really was an ulcer, "arrrhhh! well", he thought, that will clear up in a week! The week ended, the ulcer got worse, now it was bigger and pulsing and he finally looked. "OhOh!" He thought and showed his wife; "an infection", she said categorically, "Right !"said Mr Ed, "attack it with something, drain it! That will fix it!" "No! No!" said his wife, "time for the dentist", "Oh!" Said Mr Ed. Mr Ed was at the Dentist on Monday morning, thinking, "it's just an evaluation, nothing going to happen here". "It's cactus" said the Dentist, (code for major gum infection, tooth removal necessary). "No!" Thought Mr Ed, now I want to run far, far away. "I'll stay with you, hold your hand and feed you honey and tea until you are better," said his wife. "Ok!" said Mr Ed. Then every day Mr Ed got better and better.

As we saw in Chapter 1, Maslow used his pyramid to represent the hierarchy of needs human beings follow until ultimately they may be able to actualise their potential.

So, too, if we follow the "disasters in adversity" graph, choosing defence mechanisms of a less mature nature in order to avoid responsibilities in the world we don't succeed. The graphical representation shows the person becoming more and more stressed whilst making poorer and poorer decisions, eventually they go off graph altogether. Another way of representing this is in the inverse pyramid. We will become depressed and sink lower and lower in our feelings of self-esteem and self-worth. Instead of actualising we will eventually disintegrate and this is a point which we all recognise as the most extreme negative.

Everything in HR is about avoiding this

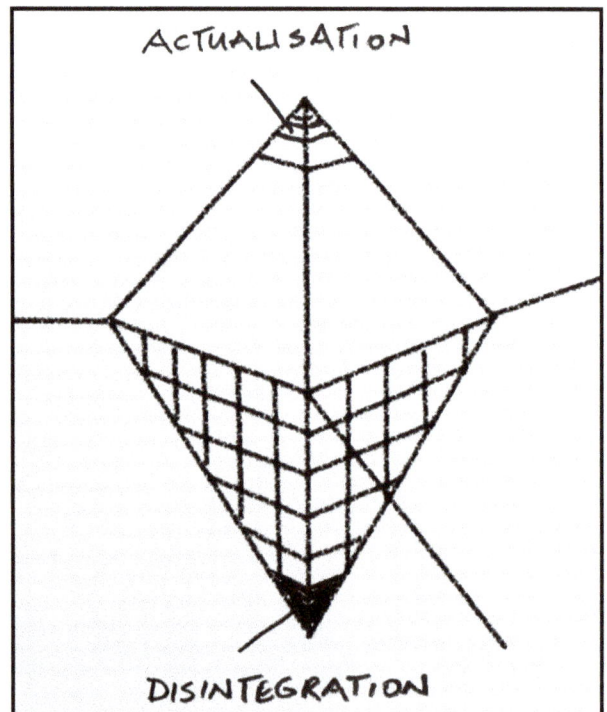

ACTUALISATION

DISINTEGRATION

and choosing a better path, one which leads us to our Centaur. Let's move on to the next two quadrants which do take us there!

Quadrants 3 and 4

The second half of the shield shows the defenses we develop as we grow and become more mature allowing us to make decisions and take independent actions leading us towards ultimate adulthood and the possibility of our Centaur.

Again this part of the shield is broken into the thoughts and feelings expressed by the Rider and the actions undertaken by the Horse. Obviously, again, these two processes are tandem, the duality of Horse and Rider being expressed synchronously.

The Rider's Quadrant

Self-Assertion entails being able to deal with adversities by having enough maturity and trust in others to realise your own issues and then being able to express those thoughts and feelings. The mature rider has developed enough self-esteem to disclose to others their feelings and experiences, having had enough positively reinforcing interactions to trust in doing this. Essentially this is about knowing that you need to tell someone you if have a problem that you need assistance with; what you feel and think about that, and helping them to understand you better, which in itself assists you with the problem while developing and reinforcing relationships and networking support systems.

For Example: A Moving Experience

Upon arrival in the strange new city, the couple looked for anything familiar and at the local shopping centre, they found a café in a bookshop. They both liked books and coffee and the shop was owned by Al and stunningly enough, as it turned out, Al came from the couple's home country!

Sitting with Al on that first day, they discussed what it was like to have moved there and how lost and disoriented they were feeling. They had already been through the overwhelmingly different obstacles and adversities just getting there, then, alone, trying to find their way round, not speaking the language and feeling very much like "fish out of water". They also talked about why they had come to the city and the plans they had for a business that they were contracted to resuscitate. Al listened and presented ideas of his own based on his experiences of living in the city for 10 years. After some weeks of daily coffees and talking, Al introduced the couple to other people who frequented his café. Many friendships were formed and hurdles were shared from the tables at Al's Café.

Mentally rehearsing possible situations and activities before doing them is something that I like to call "Imagineering". A lot of sports people use this to practice in their minds eye the moves, actions and potential game plans that they will make before they actually perform the activity. Artist's often see a picture in this same "thought space", before they capture it on canvas or in stone. Turning the subject around in your in mind and watching it unfold, assists you in practicing and mastering your imagineering of it from all of the different angles possible before you do it. Every individual HR will conceptualise their imagineering differently just as every artist perceives the essence of their vision differently.

Laura had a regular back exercise regime which included doing sets of chin ups. She knew they were the hardest but most rewarding exercise that she did. The night before doing this exercise, Laura would lie in bed with her eyes closed, imagining herself on the bar. The muscles in her back, shoulders and arms were all strong and in concert, gripping with an overhand hold and letting herself go, arching slightly, then slowly pulling her body weight up in a rowing motion, breathing rhythmically. She was as light as a feather, easily achieving her goal number of repetitions.

The next day at the gym, after stretching and mentally rehearsing the movement again, Laura's ability to do her chin ups improved markedly; she was able to do more than the previous week. A wonderful feeling of elation flooded through her with this achievement, making that day, a great one!

Self-Observation

Taking the time by making the time to meditate and really consider how you feel about a situation or issue, constitutes self-observation. Reflecting upon how you feel about it, about your motivations with reference to it and what your responses may have been already, will all assist you regarding your imagineering of how you behave in the situation. The concept of a "self-observing-ego" has been with us for years but practicing it, like meditation, is work for HR, but work which promises the greatest rewards of all.

Castles in the Air

A young woman went for a run and on that day she had two choices, she could take the bay road or the lake path. Considering this while stretching for ten minutes, she chose the bay way.

As she jogged along the path, past the boat club, she felt the first fifteen minutes of the run working at her body until she slowly began to relax the kinks out of her legs and torso. Her mind began to clear, and she let her body sink deliciously into the rhythmic movement of her Horse. It was only then that she became aware and began to consider the thought which had been nagging for relief in the back of her mind, and which she had been avoiding for some time. "I have two choices in my life right now, the teaching path or the nursing path".

As she continued her run, these two career paths stretched out before her in her mind. What was the best decision for her life? Both paths were open to her; how did she feel about each? Both paths had ups and downs and both came with the requirements of needing plenty of patience and learning. However they each had very different views of life and would produce exceptionally different experiences for her; one worked with children and the other with adults.

The young woman ran under a bridge and then began the ascent of the famously steep hill, her body slowing slightly for the task ahead, her mind now, meditatively in tune with it, working on all levels, her HR system paralleling perfectly. She was sweating by the time she got to the top. The last leg of the journey passed by a pretty little beach which small children were playing on and building a large sandcastle.

The young woman watched them while she ran along, suddenly a larger than usual wave came rushing up! The children cried out in alarm as the side of the castle dissolved back into the sea. Undeterred they examined the damage, scooped up their buckets and spades and ran laughing back to the wet sand to rebuild their fortress.

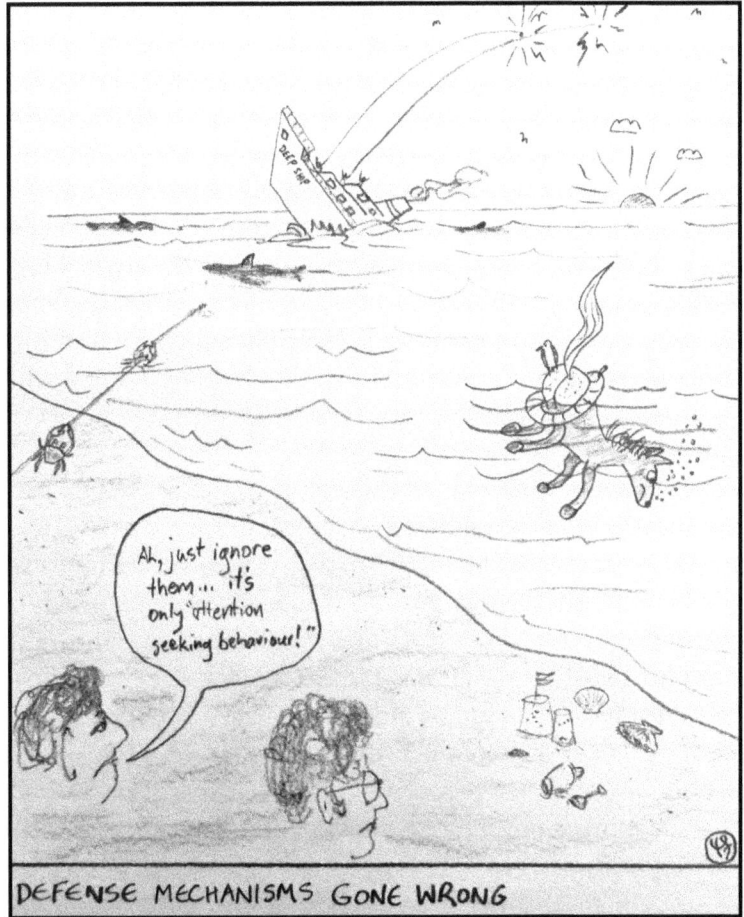

DEFENSE MECHANISMS GONE WRONG

Noticing her own reactions to the spontaneous joy in the children's play, the young woman felt her heart melt and she smiled both inwardly and outwardly "I want to be a part of that joyous being", she thought as she ran down the last hill home, racing herself, flying high, the next path was chosen!

Planning alternative solutions or responses to situations and adversity: This again is similar to my "imagineering" or visualisation. It's great to have alternative plans with which you are familiar should your first choice not work out or be showing signs that it's turning to custard! These alternatives, however, are never so magical that we can evade adversity forever by being clever, sometimes we just have to take a deep breath, as it were, and do our best with being situationally taken over.

Putting off Immediate Gratification of Rewards

This is one of the more difficult of the defence mechanisms for beginners. Today, more than at any other point in the known history of our species on this planet, we have more choices to partake in a seemingly infinite variety of "things". Immediate gratification is the philosophy projected by consumerism and delaying it seems too many, almost unintuitive! Reward, by its definition, however means something treasured, something rare and desired. To say that everything can be had immediately and without effort is oxymoronic! It's "affordable luxury". The balanced and mature HR system finds its own deeper reward within itself: the Centauring Circle produces our own magic when it is attuned and fully functional.

Humour

Every time Joe climbed into his car to travel anywhere, he was assaulted by the same thought which struck him unavoidably: that there were some cities on this planet that just seemed to not be designed for travel by road anymore and which also had a heck of a lot of people living them! The highways and byways like a tossed spaghetti floundered out before Joe; a clogged complex of buses, taxis, cars and motorbikes all emitting their own special noises and fumes, accumulating at ground level in denser and denser waves before slowly becoming the orange brown clouds blocking out the tropical sun. He was on the way to the airport to be catapulted high up above the chaos of this particular set of spaghetti streets. Would he make it? In the numerous, and yes, repetitive café discussions we had all described trying to make sense of that creeping sensation of being somewhere but getting nowhere, feeling. Many conversations flowed from this topic, that is, if we could ever make it to the Café!

In the meantime, it seemed that everything crawled by faster than Joe's car. People walking, push bikes laden with ripening produce and even cats often made better speed. Joe took a phone call, "I'm sweating" said Joe into the receiver, at his friends enquiry regarding today's traffic. Joe described the slow roasting that the journey following a mechanical fault which had taken out their air-conditioning for the last two hours had been; with the windows wound down to prevent asphyxiation in the sweltering heat, only to be greeted by partial asphyxiation from the diesel fumes billowing in the gaps, but it was at least moving. The conversation continued with the usual synopsis of topics.

Joe glanced out the window to see why today, the highway was so slow. To his mounting horror he saw signs that it was flooded still by last nights monsoonal rains and would be closed for hours yet to come. As a living part of the intestinal peristalsis of the worming traffic, his car turned slowly back into the mire of machines spread out before him; doomed, he looked up to see one of the beautiful cultural icons of the city. "I was wrong" said Joe to his friend on phone. "I'm nowhere near where I thought I was, turns out I'm just going through the Gates of Hell now!" The echo of raucous laughter was heard reverberating around AL's cafe for weeks after.

Humour is one of the most remarkably powerful defence mechanisms we have to help us in times of adversity. It can define people, moments and forge friendships that last lifetimes. It is the best medicine. No surprise then that the most loved television series are comedies. Seeing the good amongst the bad and the ugly, and being able to manifest humour from it remains one of the best defenses of all.

The Horse Quadrant

This is the final quadrant of the Centauring Circle. We see here the best defence mechanisms we can use which involve our bodies and their movements. This is the Horse at it's best and when we are able to attune these defenses to those of the Rider's in our parallel process, we open the door to being Centaured ourselves, this, then begins the experience of our Third Nature.

Turning to others for help, guidance, support, friendship: we channel this affiliation to others, allowing ourselves to be perceived by others as needing, wanting and deserving their help, guidance, support or friendship. Having this self-worth enables us to extend our experiences in adversity (life) to include wider options of responding to it. Being a part of a group that has positive identifications and which in itself operates in the wider community in healthy ways is the best of human endeavours.

Channeling Negative Feeling into Healthier Responses and Activities

Max's story: Max sat, behind his large, portable computer screen, day after day, sinking deeper and deeper into listlessness, within his growing stupor, seemingly even unable to acknowledge the patrons of his cafe. Max's girth was expanding beneath the table he sat at, it's growth the biggest movement in Max's life. Tension radiated from every pore of him whenever someone approached within a few metres; this palpable irritability successfully fended off most comers.

Fifty metres away from Max lay a sparkling, refreshing swimming pool and a further ten metres away, a fully stocked gymnasium beckoned, but it may well have been fifty years away from Max, whose narrowed gimlet eyes spied friends coming and going from either or both on their regular visits. The glue of his depression had him stuck fast to his chair and the food he was eating more and more of assisted him in staying put in his shrinking inner space.

Five years later, his friends descended to a different country, a different cafe and a wildly different Max: he jumped up to greet them, his hair cut in a modern style which suited him perfectly, his physique sharpened, svelte and strong. Max positive radiated warmth, affection, success and health! What had happened to the old Re Lax-Max, as he had been affectionately but disparagingly known by some? Max recounted his journey; watching over those years, the influence of steady and regular exercise along with a good diet had on his friends. He really worked on overcoming his internal inertia because he understood that he was missing out on his second nature. His friends were true and had offered him their company, inviting him to join them in the gym or pool at the time. Their model provided him the step by step examples he adopted in his resolution to make an active change.

He moved his cafe offshore from its origins, and worked as hard on his second nature as he had in his chair, on his business. This led him to re-discover his third nature which produced not only phenomenal changes in his HR system but Max began successfully designing cafe businesses internationally.

Having Fun/playing: Just as humour is seen as one of the best defence mechanisms we can have against everything flung at us in life, so too, naturally enough is the seemingly simply concept of having fun and playing.

We have seen in Chapter 1 that our child does not die off, our child does not go away. It is alive within us, as are all of the phases of our lives. The child, in many ways becomes subsumed by the Horse, somatised in fact. Smells, flavours, sounds and sights trigger memories remarkable for the clarity they evoke. Our child moves forward into our physical senses and savours experiences we have in the present. Fun is never far from us but we are often defended against it! Many grown-ups feel that letting their guard down and being seen to have fun or to be playing, somehow takes away from them the hard won adult-like profile they have. Being mocked and humiliated by others is a universal fear which prevents many from the single greatest emotional release available: fun and play. Adults, defended against it come the closest to it possibly, when they have sex, which is great adult fun. The HR system, when running in the positive parallel process opens to the Centaur. The Centaur, or third nature, has a fluidity of state which we will examine in much more detail in the third Chapter.

Using these diagrams and the examples given, you can start evaluating your own defensive shield and how it is uniquely operating. Let this be the first step on your journey, harmonising your HR to rediscover your Centaur. This journey will, holistically, give you better health for a longer life; one in which you will feel better, look better and comprehend your own unique and indivisible life force.

Which of these defenses do you use the most? Try to be objective as you do this, and if you are not sure, check with a close friend or relative, but make it someone who knows you well. Don't forget they have the same shield; it may rotate slightly differently, but no one misses out on having this internalised system. It operates like our lungs do, quite unconsciously until a crisis happens.

With some awareness of the use of our defenses, we can break down these quadrants and understand which are our most useful defenses for coping with the hurdles we face; our Adversity.

This is a way of understanding how the Rider affects the Horse and how the Horse affects the Rider. It is our unique and unusual duality of being; we are the Horse every bit as much as we are the Rider, and until we include both as an act of consciousness we are never truly ourselves, never truly the Centaur of our being.

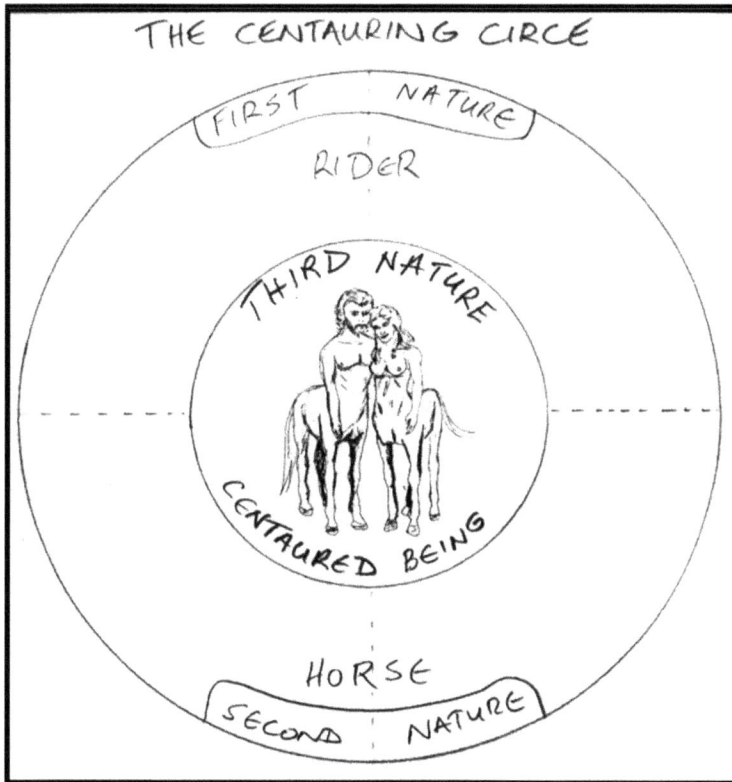

THE CENTAURING CIRCE

FIRST NATURE

RIDER

THIRD NATURE

CENTAURED BEING

HORSE

SECOND NATURE

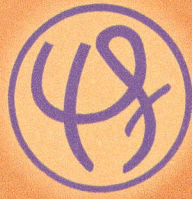

CHAPTER 3

ADVENTURES WITH ADVERSITY

*'These adventures with adversity are only really enjoyable,
if you come back from them!'*

Sara Beaumont-Connop

So! Here we are at the beginning of the journey towards our own holistic Centaur; accompanying us as guides, the defenses we have evolved to master both our internal selves, the HR duality, along with the external environment. We have seen that the doorway to our Third Nature, the Centaur of our being, lies in the conscious work of engaging our First and Second natures together as one using the higher or more evolved of our defence systems. These first two natures working in tandem potentially manifest our Centauring experience, but it doesn't happen in a vacuum. We have to locate this potential action before we can engage it, and so, now we pose the question again: "What is the meaning of adversity?"

"Adversity" is a word which conjures up many different meanings; what is an adversity to some is not experienced as such by others. However, if I use the analogy of children's board games, I think you will agree that most are based on adventures in adversity! Snakes and Ladders for instance, has the player completely at the mercy of the roll of a dice and for those of you who have played it, there is nothing worse than feeling like you were getting somewhere, only to slip down a snake to have to start all over again! As we get older, games get a bit more interesting because we are making some of the decisions, for instance: after the dice lands in Monopoly and some card games. These games are worked out in sequential steps, some being positive, some negative, and again, we don't always win! We do learn, however, that there is a better chance of us winning if we have a strategy or two; alas for those amongst us who have had a sibling that took over the bank with criminal intent!

We see in this analogy, albeit children's game's; ways in which we are rehearsing life through our child, preparing us for adult experiences. In every life experience we find the same dynamic equation searching for a balance which is contingent upon a few variables: the level and intensity of the individual's experience of adversity, along with which defenses they use to engage their external and internal realities, here is an example: Two expatriate women lived in a remote isolated area. Both of their husbands worked long hours away from home. Both women were far from their extended families and their own cultures and they had both arrived in this far flung location at the same time. During the early months of adjustment, the first woman, Judy, felt tense and irritable trying to settle into a new home and she did not speak the local language. There were misunderstandings over trying to get the house set up, she could not just run down the road to the shops in her car as every single thing had to be ordered and delivered by the local people. Judy developed headaches and felt lethargic during the day; she stayed in bed long after her husband had gone to work, the loneliness of leaving all her friends, family and culture began to sink in. By the third month she knew she needed to do something or she was not going to make it in this placement. A visiting psychologist worked with her evaluating her situation and together, they devised a plan initially focusing on getting her up and moving and out of the house. Judy started bike riding early in the morning after her husband left for work. At this time of the day she avoided the intense tropical heat and began to see the many and varied birds and animals that she had never noticed before. This activity gave her a way of exploring her new environment, including saying "hello" to people out and about along with a physical activity taking her out of the house. During this time

Judy began to think about her new life from the perspective of the limits and opportunities it presented. After this period of conscious adjustment where Judy was using the activity of riding every day to cope with the isolation, loneliness and confusion which are a normal part of living for the first time in a new culture, she decided to set up a hydroponic greenhouse and grow all her own vegetables. She combined this with studying horticulture in a long distance learning programme. It was a complicated process, however, during its orchestration Judy started to bloom in the environment! She often supplied other community members with produce and expertise in horticulture. Local people organised visits to learn how to develop their own systems and Judy was always in demand as a teacher. Her only ongoing challenge was keeping those baboons off her squash!

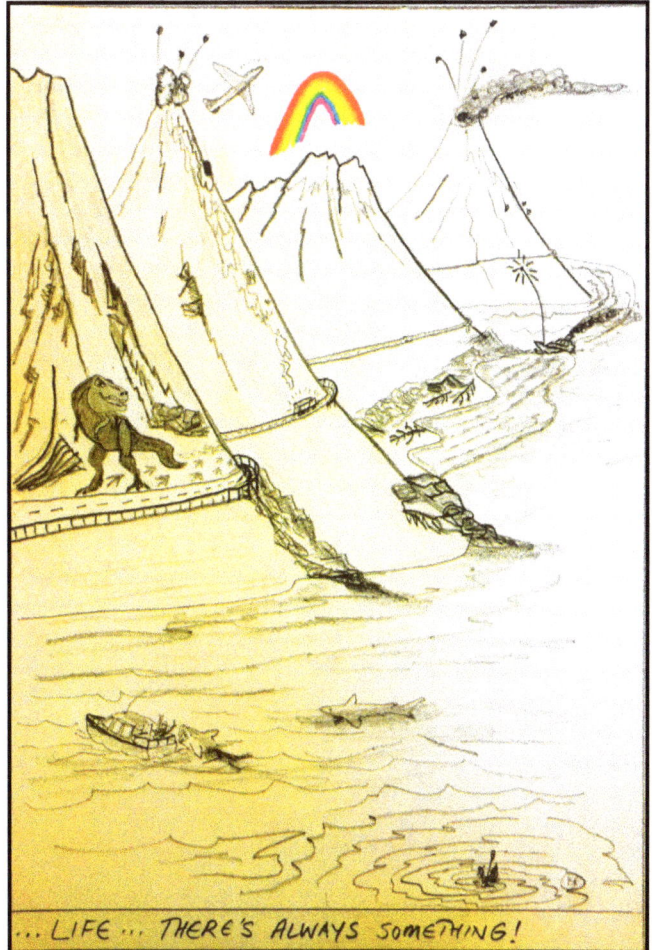

... LIFE ... THERE'S ALWAYS SOMETHING!

The second woman was Ruth. Ruth had exactly the same reaction as Judy to the sudden shock of the new culture and the equally commensurate loss of her old culture. Ruth however, decided to cope by taking the six hour bus ride to the nearest airport and then fly a further four hours to a large regional city staying in the most expensive hotel suite. She then spend a tremendous amount of money shopping for anything she felt she needed. Ruth went through tens of thousands of dollars buying unusual antiques, foods that were exotically rare and imported along with designer clothing and incredible collectables. Over time their home became a shrine to her spending and many people waited for an invitation to one of her famous dining extravaganzas where they could marvel at the extent of her excesses and wonder, privately, how the relationship she was in survived. At Christmas, the four immense and incredibly expensive Fereghan carpets dominated the living spaces. Ruth's maids furtively shopped at her house, the shelves were so full Ruth's memory could not contain the entire inventory of each and every item. Spaces could be artfully rearranged and go unnoticeable for long periods of time. Ruth's husband eventually started having angry outbursts and the marriage tension was palpable to outsiders. Ruth's weight soared as she ate the foods stacked in the larder and watched the gardeners she had hired landscape her fantasy back yard. Ruth was an almost unbearable person to be close to when she wasn't presenting her latest acquisition. These objects and events were for her, extensions of herself, without them she was empty, depressed and suicidal.

The defensive shields are in place, the external environment and the corresponding internal anxiety of major change are the adversaries. The big questions are these:

What is the change being provoked by adversity in the holistic health of these women and in which quadrants are they manifesting it?

Are there positive changes to the HR? If so, why? Are there negative change to the HR? Again, why is this occurring?

Have a look below at The Psychophysiological Signs of Adversity circle. Try to identify the various defenses being used by these two women. They are each in a reactive state of captivity to begin with, they each share very similar reactions to the deprivations they feel and the culture shock they are experiencing in fact and both of them have the HR parallel processes occurring but there are two remarkably different outcomes.

In this chapter we discuss how we can understand and harness the Horse; this whole secondary defence quadrant of ourselves. In doing so, we are gaining a mastery and balance within ourselves and the interactional environment we are in. We will develop better techniques of engaging our higher defence mechanisms that support and sustain us wherever our adventures in adversity take us and the greatest potential reward is the unfolding discovery of the Centaur!

The Signs of Adversity

We have within ourselves the single greatest resource system allowing us to gauge the adversities we may be currently wrestling with. These adversities can often actually be hidden from our conscious mind by the very defence mechanisms we are discussing. Our unconscious defence mechanisms are always attempting to insulate us from the potentially overwhelming nature of life as adversity, but in doing so can blind us to our plight; think back to how Crystal was attempting to cope. Our psychophysiological signs of distress are the gift we can use to gauge our struggle and these are the very signals of warning the centaur has to acknowledge and then act on, accessing their holistic health, examining it and developing a plan to change strategy.

Psychophysiology, our HR system of duality, provides the (self) observer with the tools to measure how the engagement with adversity is faring. There are literally thousands of well-known examples of people using their psychophysiology to overcome extreme adversity, hurdles, and life challenges, enabling them to attain goals that would never have been possible if they had just "thought about it", but did nothing; in other words, engaged the Rider but not the Horse. We have referred to Nelson Mandela's struggle to maintain not only his sense of self while imprisoned but to actively grow and thrive through it.

SIGNS OF ADVERSITY

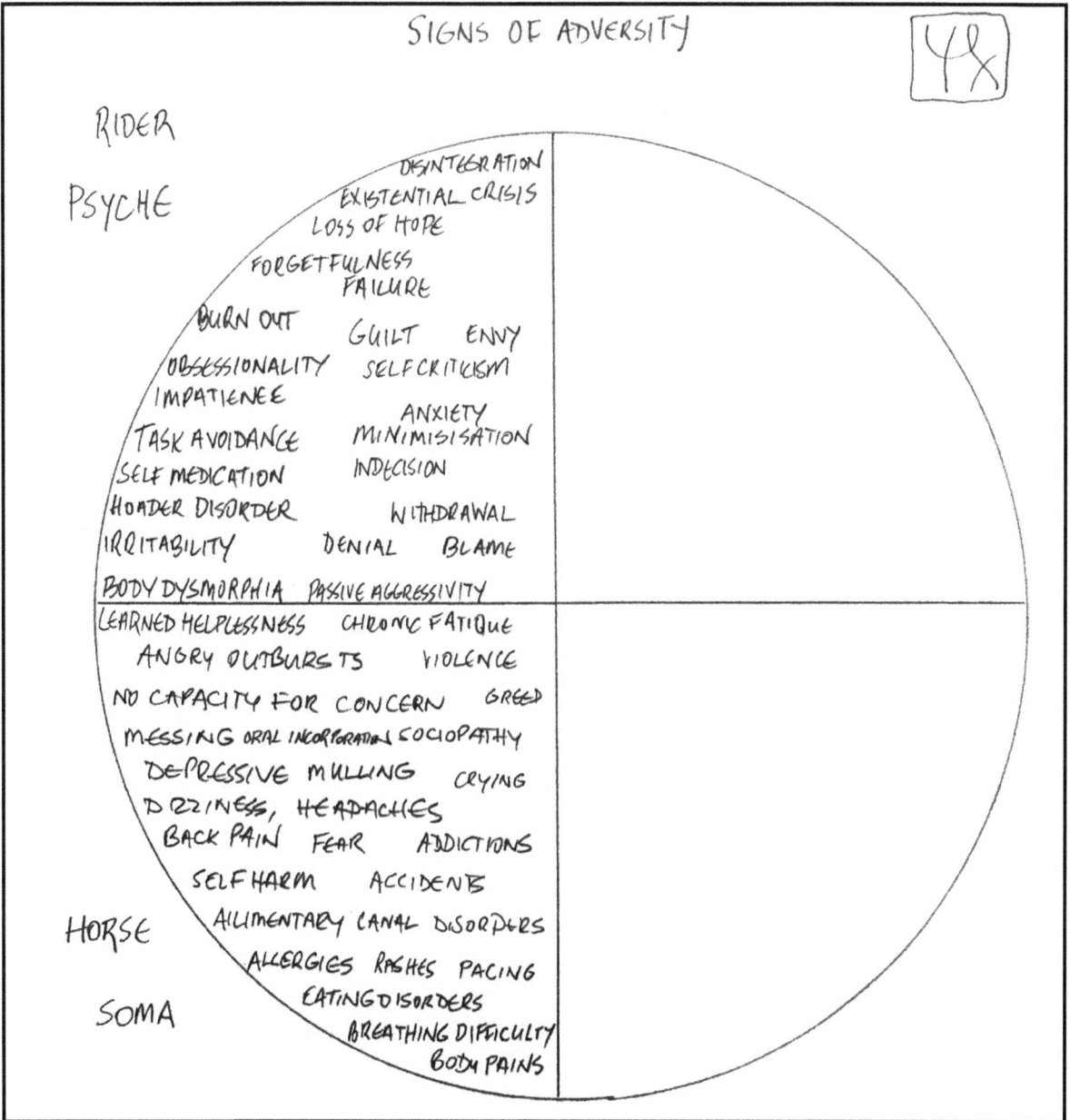

RIDER

PSYCHE

DISINTEGRATION
EXISTENTIAL CRISIS
LOSS OF HOPE
FORGETFULNESS
FAILURE
BURN OUT   GUILT   ENVY
OBSESSIONALITY   SELF CRITICISM
IMPATIENCE
TASK AVOIDANCE   ANXIETY
                 MINIMISISATION
SELF MEDICATION INDECISION
HOARDER DISORDER   WITHDRAWAL
IRRITABILITY   DENIAL   BLAME
BODY DYSMORPHIA PASSIVE AGGRESSIVITY
LEARNED HELPLESSNESS   CHRONIC FATIGUE
ANGRY OUTBURSTS   VIOLENCE
NO CAPACITY FOR CONCERN   GREED
MESSING ORAL INCORPORATION SOCIOPATHY
DEPRESSIVE MULLING   CRYING
DIZZINESS, HEADACHES
BACK PAIN   FEAR   ADDICTIONS
SELF HARM   ACCIDENTS
ALLIMENTARY CANAL DISORDERS
ALLERGIES RASHES PACING
EATING DISORDERS
BREATHING DIFFICULTY
BODY PAINS

HORSE

SOMA

In Ruth and Judy's story we see that it is only natural when any major change occurs a certain amount of denial is engaged as we try to present in the world as normally as possible, to fit in and appear alright with this new situation. Both women would have used this to initially filter their feelings of anxiety brought about by the massive change in circumstances, however we are using this example to see the divergence of responses in their individual defensive patterns.

RUTH AND JUDY COMPARED ON THE CENTAURING CIRCLE

ENVIRONMENTAL PRESSURES

OUTSIDE ENVIRONMENT

FIRST NATURE

RIDER

RIDER

(R) SUICIDAL
(R) LOSS OF HOPE/CRISIS
(R) OBSESSIONALITY, IMPATIENCE
(R) SELF MEDICATION
(R) DENIAL, BLAME, WITHDRAWAL IRRITABILITY, ANXIETY
(J) INITIAL ANXIETY, DEPRESSION
(R), (J) CULTURE SHOCK REACTIONS
(R) 'HOARDER DISORDER'

(J) SEEKING SELF IMPROVEMENT
(J) HUMOUR
(J) VISUALISATION
(J) COURAGE
(J) SELF OBSERVATION
(R+J) PLANNING ALTERNATIVE STRATEGIES

(J) EXPERIENCED MOMENTS OF CENTAURING

THIRD NATURE

(R) EATING DISORDERS
(R) DEPRESSIVE MULLING
(J) INITIAL CRYING AND DEPRESSION
(R) NO CAPACITY FOR CONCERN OF OTHERS
(R) HEAD AND BODY ACHES
(J) INITIAL HEADACHES, LETHARGY

(J) ACQUIRING NEW SKILL PHYSICALLY
(J) TURNED TO OTHERS FOR SUPPORT GUIDANCE, COMMUNITY AFFILIATION
(J) CHANNELED NEGATIVE ENERGY INTO PHYSICAL ACTIVITIES

HORSE

HORSE

ENVIRONMENTAL PRESSURES

SECOND NATURE

OUTSIDE ENVIRONMENT

SIGNS OF ADVERSITY

SIGNS OF SUCCESS

(R): RUTH
(J): JUDY

60

Ruth used obsessional and regressive behaviours as her response pattern to her psychophysiological signals. She retreated back, regressing to her child self and then bestowed upon that child a source of never ending gifts in order to make herself feel better about the situation. Ruth started to suppress her anger and fear by physically putting on weight, by armouring up with an insulation as she ate comfort food for her child self who felt abandoned and alone. She also blamed her husband for bringing her to that place and she punished him by spending the money and by alienating herself through an internal splitting away from him and leaving in her place a caricature of her former self. A repetitive motif of frustration acted out between the couple was expressed as shouting matches followed by sullen withdrawn periods and less and less frequent make up coupling as their relationship deteriorated.

Judy began to react to her experiences of adversity in the same as Ruth but differed insofar as she asked the visiting psychologist to help. Getting someone with expertise to work with her assisted Judy to engage the adversity in ways that invited creativity, physical action, social interaction locally and to use higher defence mechanisms overall. Judy had as many people lining up to visit as Ruth did but Judy's visitors emulated much of Judy's learning, taking it away and imbuing their own lives; Ruth's on the other hand were invited to envy and gossip, their take always were not positive.

Have a look at the comparison of Ruth and Judy *(opposite)* on the Centauring Circle. Graphic pictures show the principle differences in the defence styles these two women used. Similar negative experiences were shared by both women, as mentioned, but over time the differences in the quadrants was marked with Judy scoring mainly in the Signs of Success and Ruth in the Signs of Adversity.

If we refer back to the original Centauring Circle and the Psychophysiological defence diagram and think about the examples offered, it becomes obvious that if we use some of the more primary defenses to engage our adversity it follows that we are more likely to trip our horse and rider up. If we are overwhelmed by the adversity in any way there is a disconnection between our dual systems. The HR system is split and becomes either just Rider or Horse. Such a split effectively means that we are unable to continue on our journey in any holistic frame, unable to engage our First and Second Natures in harmony and this will often lead us to a Moment of Crisis. Can you remember a Moment of Crisis in your own live, a time when a change or choice had to be made? Can you remember what sparked it; was it leaving school, deciding on a job or career, leaving home or choosing to live with someone; even deciding to change a hair style can be a moment of crisis, particularly afterwards looking in the mirror. Have a look at the Levels of Adversity chart on the following page, to assist choosing one.

It is important to gain an understanding of what was going through your mind and your body at that juncture. What are the messages that travel from the library of the past to the front desk that is issuing the new books? These are the messages we stored in the saddlebags, internalised dictums often projected into us by parents, teachers and others who, at the time they yelled them at us, we're not managing their own adversities but rather dumping them on us. The Classified Section of our library can be full of these sorts of messages and in our

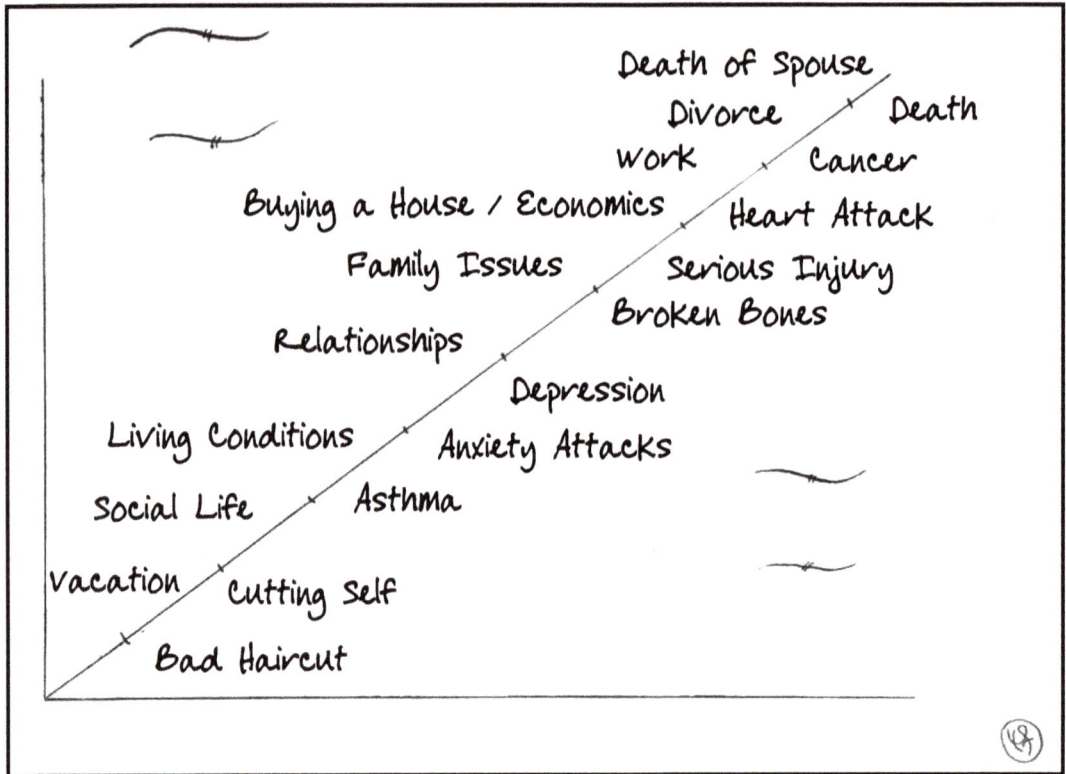

moments of crisis, when our hard fought for HR system is tripped up by adversity they can tumble out. Along with these historical messages are quite often very similar external environmental cues, cues which can trip the HR up because they mimic circumstances where we have fallen and had moments of crisis before. They can be from our familial life, from work or a social setting or simply occur in the natural world.

Reality Bites: The "External" Family

The internal world of defenses is always connected to the external world of relationships; what part do the individuals we live with and are related to play in our journeys? These people may come and go in our lives but their imprints are found in our minds and in our interactions with the world in general. Because the definition of perfect has yet to be perfected and what is normal is always debatable our family ties are a conundrum that most of us wrestle with at different times, or there would not be a flourishing trade in psychological therapies. They can be our external "greek chorus", giving advice or making judgements we don't want or need and then again, sometimes they can be the source of our greatest joys and our deepest sadness's. Being able to make good boundaries with them as adults can be difficult as we are often dragged back into feeling very childlike in our dealings with them because of the lifelong relational patterns and dynamics we have had. Having an understanding of the seesaw of relating can be very useful particularly getting to know the triggers of the child: "when do you see red?" or where is the guilt coming from? When working with children and their families in therapy we always began the first session with a picture, the picture is called a genogram, it is the pictorial story of the child and their families relating over as many generations as can be remembered by the parents; in other words a family tree. This genogram differs from a family tree in as much as we are looking for intergenerational patterns of behaviours, births, deaths, abuse, and as many of the details surrounding these events. A large amount of information is generated from this one activity and all these things have had an impact on the child's life. For example, if a child's grandfather had been in an alcoholic, he may have been violent towards his wife and children, which may have then lead to his son behaving violently towards his wife and child. If you have had a chaotic upbringing and feel it is causing difficulties in your present situation, this is the best time to seek help from a professional counsellor just as Judy did. So these intergenerational patterns can be just the sort of thing we receive internal messages from as we find ourselves in a Moment of Crisis, perhaps within one of our relationships.

Ask yourself if the relationships you are in are adding or taking away from your life? Are they balanced most of the time or on the emotional seesaw? The path towards harmonious living is not an easy one; snares and spears are often set along the way. Quote: "You can't choose your family (of origin) but you can choose your friends and mentors".

Looking back to the Moment of Crisis exercise and choosing a low level of adversity, consider what happens physically and psychologically when I say to you, "leave this book and go for a walk outside anywhere for twenty minutes." What is your immediate response? What kind of defence message are you getting? What physical feeling comes forward: tiredness, sluggishness or an irritability at the thought of stopping a task? Is it coming from the primary part of the defenses or is it coming from one of the higher defenses? Psychologically, is the message a definite "no way!" Is it a denial and blame, as in "this writer is crazy!" or perhaps an "I'll do that later" or "that does not apply to me, I don't need to do that!" as in minimisation. This thought experiment is offered both as the experiment, inasmuch as to help you to discover what some of your own defenses might be that prevent engaging First and Second Natures in parallel as well as offering you a good example of a simple exercise which will help you at any time to cope more effectively with adversity. As an aside, it's interesting to me that a man once remarked that he never had discordant conversations when he was walking with his long term walking partner because they both engaged HR to the point of Centauring.

Seeing the Wood for the Trees

Looking at some of the choices we have made in our lives and taking responsibility for them is sometimes a very difficult to do. Utmost in people's minds is the question: "Why did I do this?" It is hard to understand why we might have been relating to the world in such a way as to create the outcomes we did. We are then confronted with the question: "How can this situation be one I can change?" For many people these realisations and confrontations are challenging as they feel like they are stuck like a horse on a carousel going around and around the centre pole.

There is a contingency implicit in our interactions with the environment we live in that we have to be flexible! In previous chapters we have discussed the idea that the child's growth is dependent upon accepting changes in physicality and thought processing; for example, most ordinary adolescents don't scream they won't go through puberty because they don't want to! However they may have something to say and do about how they go through it, in contrast to what others think, particularly their parents. So too, for us, and within this chapter we will look at gaining clarity about the effects of adversity, the defenses we are best to utilise and how they operate in everyday life.

The greatest conundrum for any individual is to decide which defenses they are using, bearing in mind the fact that if they are looking for a forward movement but are using the same strategies with no change actually occurring, then the defence used is actually causing a repetitive failure to thrive situation. These repetition compulsions, as they are known, are particularly important feedback devices which we have to understand to overcome. We mentioned an intergenerational example above, in the "External Family". Repetition compulsions come in many guises and have remarkably powerful messages for us to learn from. We almost always are in the presence of one when we have the sensation or feeling of going around and around and ending up at the same place again and again.

It seems that it takes a lot to get anyone of us to change anything and that is why I have coined the phrase "The moment of Crisis or when the Centaur bleeds from a thousand cuts." When it finally comes, it feels like a moment of crisis, however it has almost invariably come about through a domino effect of our own accommodation of environmental factors and our own internal adjustments to these factors using defenses that are not competently working for us in the situation we find ourselves in. At the beginning of the book Crystal finally evaluated the overwhelming negatives and adversities surrounding every portion of her life and realised that she had "lost her footing and her way", nothing was Centaured.

We become "comfortable" with that which we have become habituated to, especially in the physical sphere and often the effort to consider and engage our physicality is so great, our First Nature incorporates "blinkering in" as a part of Second Nature!

This "blinkering" and "carousel like living" upon which a person can find themselves, leads to several defensive behaviours which are based only on letting off negative energy, much like a boiling pot lets off steam.

Smoke gets in your Eyes, Blinkering

1. Moaning about the situation, which includes protesting about having no time to do anything about it. This behaviour falls under the help rejecting complaining category as it helps the person feel that by verbalising the issues it releases the stress. It can never be anything other than a short term fix though.

2. The person blames themselves for the situation and carries the burden of guilt. While giving the person a (false) sense of control over the issues this blinkering can lead to sickness or self-harm as the person tries to gain more and more (false) control by this method. In the one of the final iterations of this defence the negative energy is repressed and stored in the physical, the Horse's saddlebags, to avoid conscious thought about it anymore.

3. Acting out or trying to control others when feeling out of control oneself. This is most noticeable with angry behaviours such as road rage, putting others down, using angry outbursts, violence or bullying to let off negative feelings. Losing one's temper over small slights, for example going from 0 – 10 on the anger scale just because your coffee arrived a little less than how you hot you wanted it!

4. The maniacal defence of trying to fend off blinkered anxiety using alcohol, prescription and non-prescription drugs.

These are only a few of the methods First Nature uses to blinker or subjugate Second Nature in the Rider's efforts to silence the Horse. By rendering the Horse silent, the Rider makes more diffuse any of the biofeedback the Horse can give the Rider which would help to effect change and engage an adversity more holistically.

We have to repeat the question we started with above: "Why would we do such things and how can we understand our motivations and take responsibility for our own actions and choices?"

Looking for a Change Reaction

When I was working with special needs children, we had a three monthly meeting for each child. A multidisciplinary team was invited to participate including anyone interacting with the child's care and their parent, if available was always present. It was called an Individual Education Plan. Each professional would have their own perspective on the holistic health of that child. Diagrammatically the child's holistic needs would be evaluated and mapped

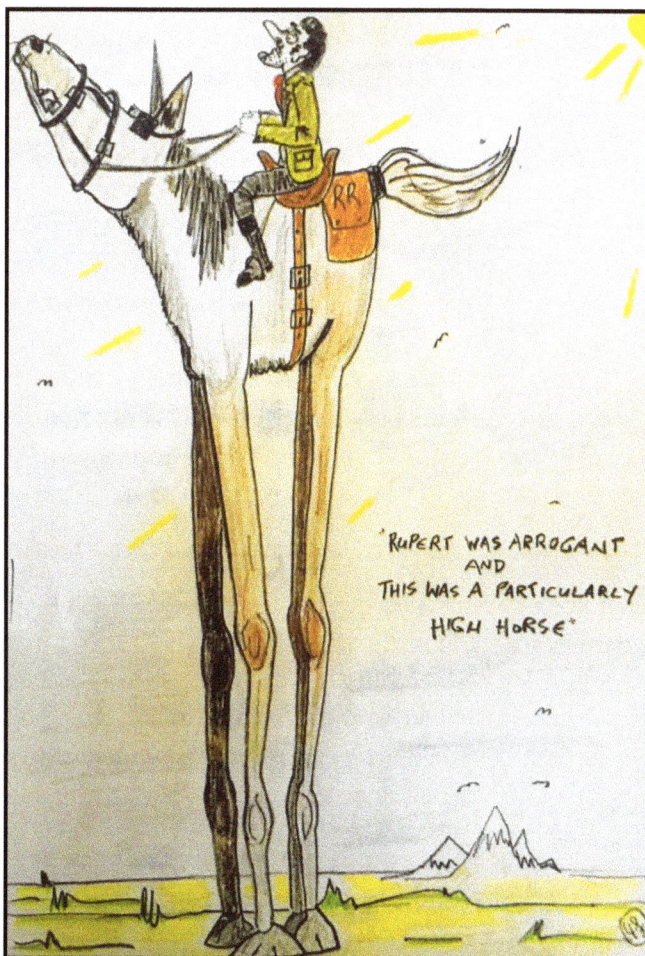

'RUPERT WAS ARROGANT AND THIS WAS A PARTICULARLY HIGH HORSE'

out; what level they were at developmentally, relationships with others, physical disabilities and so on. We then had a discussion about the changes that we wanted to facilitate in this child's life for the improvement of the Quality of it. How could we design a programme that met this child's needs on all levels? These were reviewed every three months to see what progress had been made on the previous meetings plan. We first had to decide what changes were in the best interest of the child and their family. What were the most important behavioural, learning or health issues that needed to be attended to first? These diagrams became a wheel with the child's name in the centre.

We knew we were going on a long journey with this child, they would need us to help them with many of the hurdles others take for granted, but every three month review the journey continued with the certain knowledge that quality of life is more than just existence.

Each and every one of us has our own special need for Quality of Life, most people do not want a life lying face down in faeces.

No one in Australia intentionally goes on a journey into the outback without planning that journey. There is even a television show about it called "Outback Adventures". The men presenting the show actively seek out physical and psychological challenges to pit themselves and their machines against. They have a united wisdom in planning for any of the adversities you might expect in the Outback, such as flat tyres, over heating engines, medicine kits, winches, extra water and food supplies, ropes and every kind of adaptable tool you can think of and this program has a massive following!

It is a fact that we are all unique and within that uniqueness each individual has their own special needs and deserves a plan of their own. Sometimes this fact and the individual needs are not at all well acknowledged by a society that is trying forever trying to normalise its citizens to gain a measure of control.

Given then, that we all have unique special needs, unique personal histories along with our own defence styles based on these histories, saddlebags, classified sections coupled with the unique external demands from our families, workplaces, friends, lovers and the environment itself we can begin to formulate plans as in "All Aussie Outback Adventures".

Short Term Goals in Adversity

Intrinsic to the Horse and Rider theory is the fundamental concept that key to any successful engagement with adversity, there must first exist an holistic balance and accord within our Natures in reference to the external reality.

Let's focus on holistic Centauring and the development of goals and consider why doing this may be important to you.

There are three inter-connectors of the adversity experiences that you will have probably already divined for yourself and we all have them at our disposal.

1. **Hindsight:** that is, looking back upon other situations of adversity or the one just experienced and gaining a different and more objective perspective. This is effectively using our second

nature, by understanding the impact of the adversity upon the body. This corresponds to the Horse and we often say things like "I could kick myself for not...."

2. **Insight:** follows Hindsight and allows us to gain understanding and knowledge by evaluating the conditions around the situation under which circumstances like tiredness, illness, anger, anxiety and not planning ahead may have played a part. This corresponds to the Rider.

3. **Foresight:** Following on from Hindsight and consequent Insight: The ability to learn from previously experienced situations and adapt new ways of behaving by using the newly understood insights to avoid or modify our previous understandings or "blinkered thinking" and not repeat history over and over again.

These Three Sights, provided to us through our inter-connected Natures can only be their most effective when they are holistically functioning. We can only apprehend our multidimensional being in this reality by means of Centauring ourselves harmoniously. It is very ironic that when we are in our Third Nature, the Centaur, we are quite a-temporal, that is, unaffected by time; yet in our Second Nature, Horse, we manifest as an organic being which is affected by time, and in our First Nature, the Rider, we are in between times, conscious and affected while also able to be unconscious and unaffected. This is the way of the HR, we saw in Chapter 1 why we were in this configuration and how the process of moving into our lives and the natural experience of adversity that it brought cost us. The saddlebag systems that our HR duality provide us with enabled us to move into life and to adapt as best we could. This saddlebag system however needs conscious acknowledgement and activity to process its contents or else it, in the end overwhelms us in tandem with the external demands of reality and we end up experiencing moments of

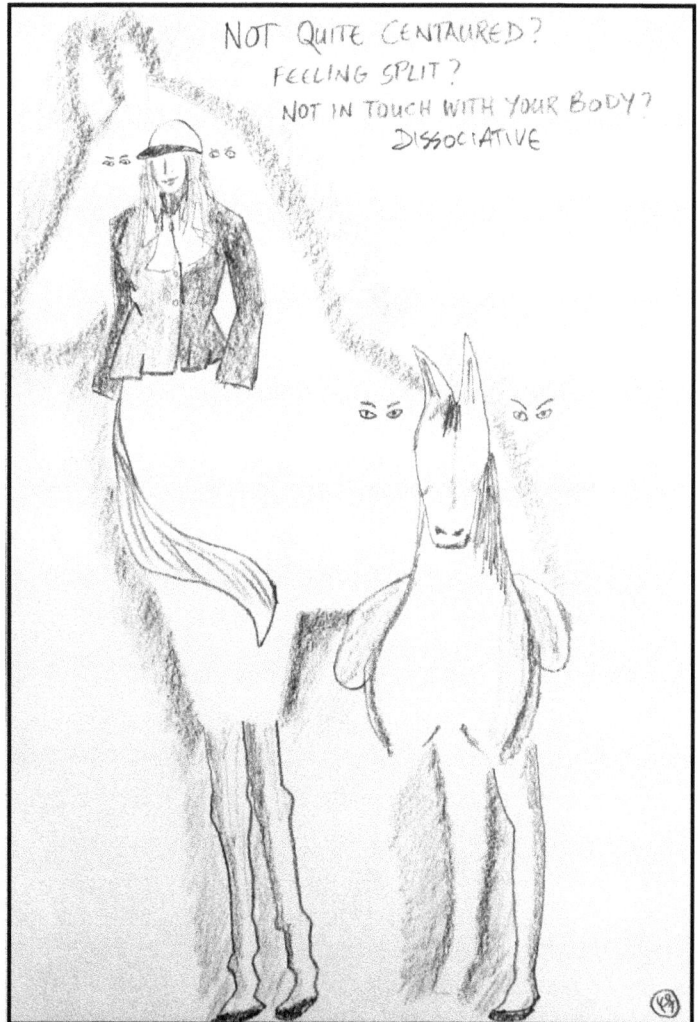

crisis. Planning and using our higher defenses consciously is the only way to engage ourselves in the World if we are to minimise moments of crisis and maximise our successes.

Let us be clear that much of what we do in life as an adult is a CHOICE, even doing nothing is a choice! We make a choice getting up in the morning or staying asleep, going to bed at night or staying awake and everything in between these hours. If we break down what we are doing, we see that we are making conscious and unconscious choices, unless someone really does have a gun at our head. Choices often evolve into habits, and until we decide to change the routine for any reason, we will not break out of the habit! One of the best ways to break out, is to go on holiday as it's "Free" time: anything can happen time.

Ben once decided to have a two week Christmas holiday where nothing was planned, everything was 'up in the air', he was free, light as a feather. The fates would smile down upon him and make something magical and exciting happen, just because he wished it so!

The first holiday morning Ben awoke, everything was quiet, all his flat mates were away camping. Ben waited, he waited all day, he watched TV, played a video game, went to the corner store, went home, watched TV again, ate and went to bed late. Every day of that two week holiday Ben awoke, hoping for adventure or at least difference, but each day the silence of indifference greeted him and finally he realised, "Hope" was not a holiday plan and being at home was not an Adventure - only a legend in his own mind!

Unlike our woe-begotten friend Ben, most of us try to plan holidays and we do map out where we would like to go. We do make short term goals for the journey. Why do we do this?

Start to think about what prevents you from choosing to change, think about the defenses you use. Ben used magical thinking, a kind of fantasy along with denial and passive aggressive defenses to deal with the anxiety of having to make a choice and plan for his holiday. In a way, he had regressed to a childlike state, hoping someone would somehow save him from his tower of boredom; reminiscent of a particular fairy tale: sleeping beauty. Psychophysiologically, his Horse and Rider lay down in his stable and waited for rescue, a common malady.

However... ***"The downside of a Circle is Up!"*** *Sara Beaumont-Connop*

Making a Difference Makes a Difference

Any movement that you make in the world at all can elicit a different response from that world! Try putting a new picture up on your wall or changing your hair style; even walking on a different path on a sunny day. A certain level of energy flow changes as you consider difference from another angle or two. It may be enough to change the kinetics of negative energy to positive.

There was once a childhood game based on an origami paper folding exercise which was called "Which number do you pick?"

A child would make a paper circular origami soothsayer, a fabulous folded paper device constructed of many multifaceted flaps. On the top of the flap were numbers and underneath were written in childish hand proclamations orders to do things or think things. Some of these orders were good, some not so good, it was a bit like the old magic 8 ball game. Anyway, everyone who was eight years old lined up to take their chances. This game had the potential to light up faces or to cause great disappointment! Just being a part of this activity, however, was to be a part of a magical energy flow from child to child. This one little messaging game made some very interesting differences.

Sometimes in our first nature we can play this game; wake up and pick a number: look under the flap and the energy changes accordingly. Think, for example about your energy on Monday morning as compared to your energy on a Sunday morning.

Baby Steps: Planning a Change, not just Hoping for One

When we embark on a holiday to a foreign land, we would like to get where we are going without getting lost or sick and have enough money, clothes and supplies to have a reasonably good time when we get there. So how would you do that for other goals you may have?

Remember that making a move in any direction can make a difference.

Talking about it is the first movement in fact, it's a type of stretching for the mind. Mind stretching is using creative imagery to engage the planning mode, an imagineering of the possible. Active discussion is best undertaken as we have seen while walking. The walking talk helps more than you might believe, to assist your mind engaging the ideas and thoughts.

This HR movement; Mind and Body stretching together actively assists the mapping of the objectives on your way to achieve the goals you have set. Clearly and realistically select choices and options that you can do, as opposed to those that are not possible.

Rehearsing what it is you want to change or achieve helps you to stay focused and motivated on the steps you need to accomplish en-route to your goal. Given that we have seen over and over again, that better outcomes are achieved from the use of the higher defence mechanisms, it is these that we obviously need to be utilising as much as is possible.

Planning Alternative Solutions or Responses to Adversity

Learning to read is full of helping the child plan alternative ways of seeing words in sentences, in stories and songs. It's about how to sound words out and which strategies to use when learning to spell a word. To gain this knowledge we all went through those early reader stepping stones.

Breaking down an activity into smaller steps is how we learn every skill we have learnt. They all have Psychological and Physical components. Let's match up the kind of higher defenses that are used when developing skills and ultimately achieving goals.

Planning for Adversity: An Example Using Ourselves

They say travel broadens the mind, well it certainly began to teach me a thing or two about

PLANNING IN ACUTE ADVERSITY

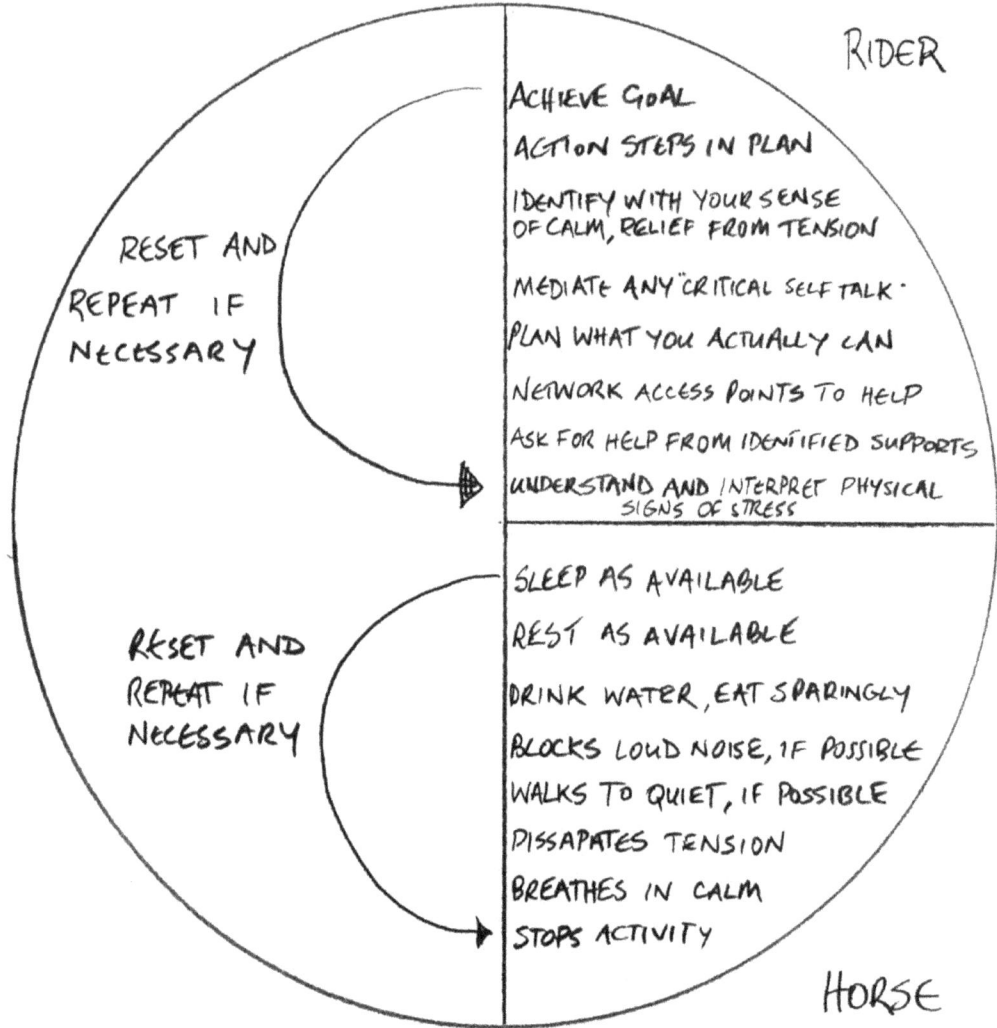

RIDER

RESET AND REPEAT IF NECESSARY

ACHIEVE GOAL

ACTION STEPS IN PLAN

IDENTIFY WITH YOUR SENSE OF CALM, RELIEF FROM TENSION

MEDIATE ANY "CRITICAL SELF TALK"

PLAN WHAT YOU ACTUALLY CAN

NETWORK ACCESS POINTS TO HELP

ASK FOR HELP FROM IDENTIFIED SUPPORTS

UNDERSTAND AND INTERPRET PHYSICAL SIGNS OF STRESS

RESET AND REPEAT IF NECESSARY

SLEEP AS AVAILABLE

REST AS AVAILABLE

DRINK WATER, EAT SPARINGLY

BLOCKS LOUD NOISE, IF POSSIBLE

WALKS TO QUIET, IF POSSIBLE

DISSAPATES TENSION

BREATHES IN CALM

STOPS ACTIVITY

HORSE

SIGNS OF SUCCESS

researching and planning for where you are going and what you might find when you get there!

My husband and I have been gifted with many opportunities to travel, however one of the most recent was to live outside our culture and really experience an integrative journey that came ten years ago.

We were looking for a new challenge in our lives, something outside the square and leafing through the Australian Saturday edition newspaper over coffee, a large advertisement for Spies caught our eyes. Two therapists could do that, we thought excitedly, after all we're paid observers and we listen for information about people..."Hazzah!" However, upon a small amount of reflection we realised our ability to speak languages other than Australian and New Zealand would put a bit of a damper on our ability to spy well! Anyway after that initial rush, we read a smaller notice underneath the larger one: Therapist wanted to run an Expatriate Counselling Service in South East Asia. "English speaking." We could do that, that we could do! Applying was done with a fair amount of light hearted disbelief that it would ever happen, that is, relocating to another country that had a totally different culture, customs and language, the works. However, fortune favours the brave and we were given an interview, commonly referred to as a "look see" in expat circles. The travel was paid for, we had four days to look around at the clinic, the city and the environment. This was a very Marco Polo moment for us, being completely foreign to this part of the world. I learned one word to go with: "Thank you". I figured manners maketh the woman and it couldn't hurt to be polite, no matter how confused we might get. Well, they forgot we needed a Visa organised so we didn't get out of the airport for a day and at every juncture I managed to mangle the language with my version of "Thank you", every official looked bemused, but stamped the forms. Our driver, waited, sign in hand, in the middle of what seemed to be a sea of others all pressing forward, touting for trade, shrouded in a haze of tobacco smoke and heat. The ride into town through the Asian mystery felt unreal. We floated past brown and green paddies, stilted platforms with a few locals adorning them watching the snaking line of traffic from airport to city; the distant past meeting the present and future of this very populous place. So it was that two, ever slightly naïve Antipodeans made the voyage into uncharted territory, Magellan-like in their curiosity, we had no idea!

It was part of our brief to help other new-comers cope with this environment. While we had both previously lived outside our cultures for some years, these experiences had been, by comparison, easy as they were still based in cultures similar to our original and had English as a first or close to first, language. So we had our own Everest to deal with; breaking down the experience into small steps became critical to everyday planning. Here are some of our issues that led to short term goal planning in a big way!

Physical Challenges

The heat was a constant 33 degrees every day and the attendant humidity close to 100%. Air conditioning that could not or would not work effectively and regular intermittent power cuts thrown in for good measure. Sleeping in the heat was very difficult and the whine of the dengue carrying mosquitos didn't help. Physically attempting to use the city environment to go for a walk or bike ride was unsafe, apart from the absolute clutter of the narrow streets with traffic going in any direction including head on with no apparent rule following other than the bravest or most aggressive driver being given right of way, there were no footpaths. Everyone either had a car, a variety of smaller four wheel drive or a scooter and they were everywhere. There were millions and millions of them which were licensed and millions more which were not. Traffic jam after traffic jam from 5am onwards, particularly Monday to Saturday were the norm and traveling to more than one destination per day within the city was near impossible. You could catch a bit of a break on Sunday till around 10am. There are large drains to contend with as well as pollution particulates in the air; "breathe in, breath out!" Any room on what might pass for a sidewalks is taken up with parked vehicles, vendors and other people just cruising and it's always 33 degrees still! There is one park in the whole city and again there is the heat and at 9am bus loads of people arrive to walk there. Biking means travelling by car to the "country", some hours out of the city and you must start early in the morning and only on Sunday otherwise the return through the traffic jams morphs into eight or more hours of sitting and waiting in traffic, without the convenience of any roadside bathroom facilities! Tennis and golf are available, however again, see heat and traffic issues. Finding foods for health in a place that has many different styles of food preparation and cooking could also be challenging and relying on café foods led to a fair few stomach issues in our first few months of residence. Last, but by no means least we're those mosquitos which loved the heat and with the open drains helping to breed batches of them, well...they love dawn and dusk and dark clothing along with warm blooded mammals and they came complete with dengue and malaria.

Psychological Challenges

The inability to speak the local language accurately led to a lot of misunderstandings: I was ordering a coffee, trying to say "no sugar" but apparently I was saying '"no crazy". We relied on the good will of our driver, who navigated and negotiated virtually everything for us in the first 6 months. We felt reduced to kindergarten level, we could not drive anywhere without him, we could not have a conversation with locals without him, we did not know where anything was without our guide and guru driver. We were totally reliant on local goodwill for help with life generally and we were the ones supposed to help the 'newcomers!

Having no social network, arriving without many contacts and being strangers in a strange land can be very isolating. No family or friends to talk to or spend time with does add a certain eerie quiet to life. It also inhibits the chances of doing anything outside the home and so it can become like the life lived on the head of a pin and you are revolving in a tiny circle around it. Culture shock, as it is famously discussed, is not so much about the culture you are propelled into at full speed, it is often more about the culture that you have left behind! Obviously the new culture and external environment that we have been talking about is stunning to say the least but the friends, walking tracks, signs, foods and water you don't have anymore can quite overwhelm the newcomer.

Cultural Differences, or, When in Rome... Do as the Romans Do

Learning from the locals what and how their local customs are and work does help enormously with better relating generally. So, my clothing went from knee length to ankle length, my shoulders and arms became covered. Everybody greets you all the time, everybody! I once said "hello" two hundred times in one day; I kept a tally. It's a polite city, what could I do?!

The psychological impact of the traffic was felt by everyone, locals and expats alike; sitting for hours in a vehicle never knowing how long it was going to take and whether you would make it at all was very frustrating and stressful. Six hour journeys were quite normal with no bathroom stops, no way out of that sweltering metal box on wheels and no information or reason why the traffic was doing whatever it was doing! One trip a day was all most people could accomplish, unless on a scooter, however the way the locals got around on those meant that there was no shortage of serious accidents, sadly.

Then there was dealing with security staff everywhere, checking usually for secretly planted under vehicle bombs, professional parkers and for many expats their live-in maids, cooks and gardeners.

Please refer to the chart on the following page, where we have used this experience to illustrate our Adventures in Adversity.

NB: It should be noted here that when faced with adversity and changes of some magnitude that a regression to a more child-like helplessness is not uncommon and seeking help is a necessary adjunct to these experiences.

Self-Awareness and the Higher Defence Mechanisms

"Where's Wally?"

It is so easy to be lost in the maze of the Horse to be asleep on the Horse, seemingly hiding from consciousness and seemingly seeking unconsciousness. We all can drift toward this state when we are saddled with a set of circumstances. A change reaction can only occur when moments of clarity are experienced in self-awareness, our First Nature thinking. The actual realisation for the need of change in response to being saddled with a set of circumstances, is a golden moment and not to be lost. It is garnered from the game of Hide and Seek that our conscious and unconsciousness minds play with each other throughout our lives. It is easy to fall asleep on the Horse as it goes through the motions of life and gets lost in the maze of everyday living. Finding the internal, and then external mirror of self-reflection can give us a more accurate picture, which can then allow us to create a decision and base our change reactions on it. Have you ever seen the children's books known as "Where's Wally?" These

ADVENTURES IN ADVERSITY			
	Adversities	Positive Actions	Outcomes
Rider **Psychological**	ISOLATION BY DIFFERENCE DANGEROUS TRAFFIC INFANTILISION LOSS OF CONTROL CULTURE SHOCK LOSS OF LANGUAGE LOSS OF HOME ISSUES WITH TRUST	JOINED EXPAT GROUPS DROVE OFF PEAK LEARNED FROM OTHERS LEARNED CULTURAL APPROPRIATENESS AND LANGUAGE SKILLS PHONED HOME DEVELOPED NETWORKS	STARTED TEACHING OTHERS DEVELOPED INCREDIBLE FRIENDSHIPS AND BONDS. IMPROVED THINKING OUTSIDE OF THE SQUARE. DISCOVERED NEW PATHS INTO FRIENDSHIPS BEYOND OUR CULTURAL NORMS
Horse **Physiological**	COULDN'T WALK ANYWHERE FOOD POISONING DEHYDRATION ISSUES RADICAL CLIMATE CHANGE DENGUE, MALARIA ETC DIFFICULT TO FIND QUALITY FOOD AND GOODS HOME SICKNESS	JOINED A GYM AND GOT A TREADMILL AT HOME. REDESIGNED WHOLE DIET. CHANGED CLOTHING AND TOOK WATER EVERYWHERE. GOT DEET AND SCREENS. NETWORKED SUCCESS. TRAVELED AND EXPLORED.	DEVELOPED EXCELLENT PHYSIQUE AND FITNESS. INVENTED A NEW PROTEIN POWDER FOR TRAVEL. ROLE MODELS FOR OTHERS. LEARNED NEW LANGUAGE AND DISCOVERED NEW FOODS. TRAVELED A LOT.

are based around trying to find a small cartoon man whom has been secreted in a mélange of environments designed to hide him well. The reader has to find Wally in the midst of the many crazy shapes and objects he hides within, only then can you colour him in and all is revealed! We have all played puzzle games of one sort or another, jigsaws, word games, arithmetic, app based and computer games, chess and at our very beginning often simple block games. They are the learning tools that schools use for the development of lateral thinking; essentially thinking outside of the square. Some friends related a tale of brilliant bargain suitcases they found while traveling a distant land. They wanted to upgrade but keep their large suitcases for another future trip. The two of them could not decide how to manage this on their "one suitcase per traveler" budget. Dumping one good large suitcase and force feeding the new smaller one everything it had previously carried, the two of them made their way home. Once there, some weeks later, she said to him: "why didn't we think to simply put the brilliant smaller ones inside our large ones and just pack around them?" "Oh", he groaned, stunned and regretful; "I guess, we just didn't think outside of that square!"

Once we have the internal-external mirror awareness, have tested some decisions and shaped them into a plan, using as much lateral thinking as we need and then added to the ingredients: self-responsibility and some commitment; we're ready to go. Joining a gym as an activity for instance, is not the same thing as using the gym. Considering the fact that it took you two years to learn to walk, using all of your higher defenses, along with your parents help, why do some people think it will only take 30 minutes of turning up and sitting on a stationary bike, looking at a screen, to change their whole physicality?

It does take intent, focus and a belief in yourself that you can achieve your goals through your plan. You need to get help from the appropriate people and develop a commitment and faith that it will slowly improve as you practice your intention. It is exactly the same process that you did as you walked and talked and grew into who you are now. Choosing an activity with which to make your life change and being able to enjoy it while you do it, gives motivation to continue and inspiration to try new things. This seems to be especially true when it is done with a partner or a group which creates a dynamic sharing of the incredible positive energies of achievements!

Defence mechanisms have evolved as an integral part of the HR system to block out or minimise the otherwise overwhelming signals of adversity and life tasks that are continually bombarding us every day. They allow us to manage what we need to manage and succeed with the adversities and tasks we engage with by the necessity of our living. The issues we have with defence mechanisms is that although they function at their best to do this, we can lose our focus and motivation in our lives and then drift, trancelike into the arms of the lower defenses like denial, minimisation and rationalisation and in a way "give up". Some of this "giving up", you will remember, is the toll we pay to pass through life as measured by the weight and toxicity of our saddlebags! The defence mechanisms in a way mirror the positive-negative pull of this universe we inhabit, as nature does abhor a vacuum. For every negative space there is an equal and opposite positive to match it, for every light matter there seems to be an equal and opposite dark matter! Recognising this "pull", or drift from focus, actually occurring within ourselves by using hindsight, insight and foresight in the way we have been describing, gives us a chance to choose opportunities that these sights can develop and then lead the way to greater self actualisation and experiences of Centauring.

Jeff was a young man, only 33 years old, he was managing a demanding business, and he was tired, dark circles underscored his eyes. Every day he felt a pain in his side from a rare, mosquito driven hepatitis picked up on adolescent adventures in the Western Pacific, leaving him with a deteriorating health. He doggedly fought to keep his job and himself afloat as he slowly sank under the weight of this illness. The Specialist he was sent to after the Physician monitoring this deterioration for a year gave up, said to Jeff to eat and drink whatever he liked, because six months was all he had left of his life, unless the Interferon worked or a liver transplant became possible! So at 33 years of age and crucified by his health, Jeff limped home to a relationship with a partner who was, because of her own fears, deep in denial about his health; no help there, he thought.

Jeff's best friend Bob had been watching this train wreck from the sidelines, he pulled his friend aside after work one day and said: "Come on Jeff", you are having an intervention, let's make a rescue plan. Bob organised an alternative health plan with Jeff, they looked holistically at Jeff's health, choosing to look at his diet first, and a radical detoxification process occurred. Jeff's liver actually started to respond to this treatment, and he lost 25 kilograms! They began a walking-talking programme which grew into an exercise regimen with aerobic and strength training on a 3 times weekly basis. Jeff moved forward with the renewed energy of this psychophysiologic process; he started his own successful business, got his younger ideal physicality back and his life became more balanced overall. Jeff even experienced Centauring moments and has stayed on the path ever since.

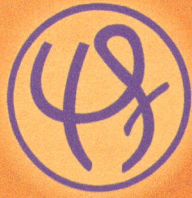

CHAPTER 4

FOOD FOR THOUGHT
- THE EXISTENCE OF EATING; EATING FOR EXISTENCE -

'Nutrition: Energy In, Energy Out'

There is a stage in every child's infancy that is hall marked by the "Peek a Boo" game played when the adult puts their hands over their eyes and then uncovers them quickly, surprising the child as if they were "popping up out of nowhere"; next, various squeaky toys are added to the game to the growing delight of the child. The infant will throw a toy or object down and away and at first not bother to look for it as it "is gone"! Then, when it is handed back, then the game continues and gradually the child's brain-hand-eye co-ordination link together to play the game in synch. The fast developing infant tumbles to the momentous realisation that just because they can't see the toy does not mean it does not exist and further, that if it is looked for, it can be found and continues its existence in the world!

The funny thing about this concept of object constancy is that when it comes to food we have an abstract conundrum: The food disappears into our internal self and we obviously lose sight of its existence, however we have an awareness that some kind of magical alchemic organisation is occurring inside us as the food is becoming US we become the food! Object constancy has transmuted from "things in the world" to an experience introjected into self. Do we make it "all gone" magically for our inner child, or can we, consciously in the moment, understand that we have added it to ourselves? It is interesting to note that we were eating in the womb before we were breathing in this external environment, such is the primacy of ingestion!

Because this is such a primary activity, a survival mechanism; and it is repeated at least 3 times a day, it is not easy to see this unique metamorphosis occurring the further away from childhood we get. Children's growth is a visible, measurable and remarkably fast physical manifestation which is acknowledged as natural, in fact, healthy. We get worried when it is not manifesting in this way! What happens to the food when we have done with our growth spurts? What does our adult physically require? In historic times food did literally mean fuel for physical labour.

Learning how to make the most of our psychophysiology can be confusing. As living beings, we are a complex bio-electro chemistry set with an equaling complex energy system. It is rare to be taught about the quality and quantity equations of food in versus energy out.

Children are encouraged to eat and grow. The meaning of Food is tied very much into the meaning of Love, care and comfort hence the term "comfort food", often used in winter cooking magazines, or following an emotional letdown.

Now that we have become quite familiar with the operations of our defence systems, particularly the qualitative difference between the higher and lower ones and we are conscious that our child-self is very much alive and subsumed into our physical being we can consider the following: "Whenever we eat, the intrinsic meaning of each meal can be feeding different parts of our self, our psychophysiology, our Horse or Rider, dependent upon our mood, body chemistry and whatever external adversity we may be facing."

Eating for Two

Once upon a time, at 8pm on a balmy evening in the topics, a friend dined with a well to do couple and their 6 year old daughter. Miss 6 and the adult friend were seated together on one side of the rather large dining room table. A special seafood meal had been ordered, and they were awaiting its home delivery. In the meantime the adults were making small talk, the child was seated entranced in a bag

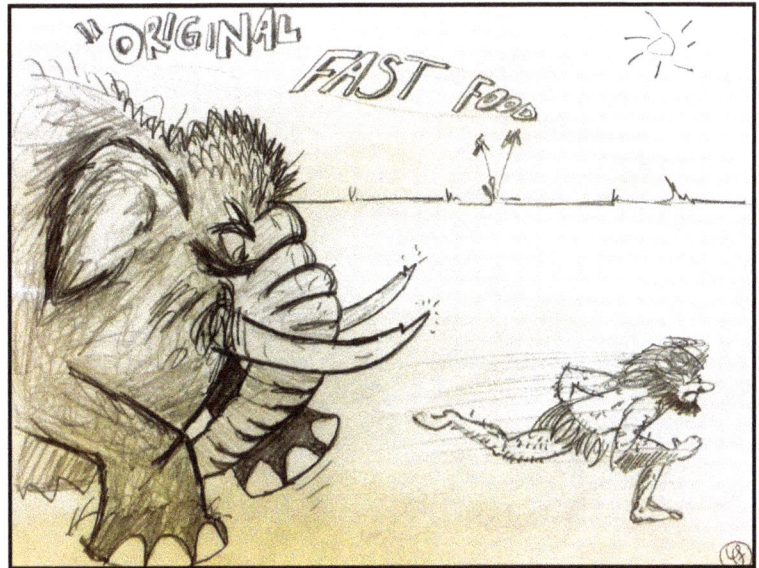

of sweets she was hungry, it was 8pm adult time, 20 past midnight child time. Methodically she consumed each pastel rosette and after about 10 minutes of nonstop consummation, the father mandated that the child's chewing cease but the girl never batted an eyelid, she just kept staring down into that bag of bright balls, passing one after another hand to mouth with great concentration, completely ignoring all and sundry! The friend meanwhile had been watching with some fascination as events were unfolding, and at this juncture of parental dictate, the friend, well-meaning but ignorant, decided to take the foolhardy action of removing the bag of sweets from Miss 6. The child reacted with an immediate and severely savage bite; the Horse had Spoken, it was Eating for two!

Knowing what's in our Food, and what it is Doing to our Physiology

Looking at the equation of Food as Fuel that the individual's physiology needs versus the individual's psychological cravings, we ask ourselves which part of our self are we feeding? For example: if your car needs a tank of gas to get to work for a week, would you keep filling your tank and pay for twice the amount you actually need at the gas station? Yet each day we eat, and in eating, are often feeding the different needy parts of ourselves directly related to how we feel. We have no plan or knowledge as to how much energy we expend; at least with the car, fuel overflows on to the ground so we know it's too much!

The psychophysiologic system we run is far more complicated than the black and white car analogy. We manifest as that duality of HR, with a mind-body that enables us to go back to the magical thinking defence of "out of sight out of mind", so it no longer exists! Our Child has spoken and the object constancy we have developed disappears just as we magically make the food disappear inside of ourselves.

So, back to the earlier question, the equation of food as fuel: how do we know what we need for our own physiology? The excess or overflow goes into our incredible storage systems, the saddlebags. It does not go there all at once but incrementally. Remember, we did not have an enormous meal once that took us from 0-20 years overnight! We are an adaptive animal that uses food as a major coping strategy psychophysiologically.

Rewarding Behaviours

Being in adversity brings out the neediness in the Horse and Rider, the physical and the psychological and it is seen nowhere more clearly than in the ways we eat and drink to feed both.

Mapping the journey you take with food each day, helps you to understand your individual psychophysiological needs best. Why do you eat and drink what you do and when you do? Are there any intergenerational patterns? When we are children, our parents fed us at various times and in various ways with typical foods and drinks, these now have a bearing on the habits of today, they are still within us as part of our natures.

Looking at the First and Second nature what does eating represent to you?

For survival
To keep warm
To feel less anxious
To feel full and content
To taste and savour
To feel safe
To feel less hurt
For health
To feel less lonely
For energy
Social opportunities

The Commercial Contrivance

The commercial world funds and closely follows research regarding our psychophysiological systems, particularly respecting how we respond and behave to certain stimuli. Their advertising is designed to capture our attention using every possible nuance and aspect of our remarkable sensory systems: sight, sound, taste, smell and touch. Careful attention has been paid to enticing the consumer into the repetitive consumption of products.

THE COMMERCIAL CONTRIVANCE AT A SHOPPING MALL NEAR YOU				
SIGHT	SOUND	SMELL	TASTE	TOUCH
COLOURS, ADVERTISING, NO OUTSIDE WINDOWS, PICTURES, TEXTURES. FOOD AND GOODS ARE MIXED AND FILL YOUR VISION IN ALL DIRECTIONS. NO EXTERNAL ENVIRONMENTAL STIMULI. IT IS CONTAINED LIKE A CASINO. NO INFORMATION ABOUT INGREDIENTS. EYE LEVEL FOODS LIKE CANDY.	MUSIC, MUSIC EVERYWHERE SOOTHING AND PUMPING. ADVERTISING NOW ALLOWED IN WASHROOMS. CACOPHONY OF COMPETING SOUNDS VYING FOR YOUR ATTENTION IN EVERY SHOP.	COFFEE, FRESH BREAD, FOOD GLORIOUS FOOD. CAFES ARE MIXED WITH RETAIL FOR MORE FOOD CALMING SMELLS MASSAGE OILS NAIL CARE CALLS	FREE SAMPLES ADDICTIVE SUBSTANCES ARE ADDED, SUGAR, FATS, SALTS, ALCOHOL LESS DEFINITION OF FOOD COURT MEANS YOU CAN EAT ANYWHERE. DRINK WITH THE HAIR DO, NAIL DO MASSAGE DO.	ALL WRAPPED IN PLASTICS. SELF HELP. CROWDED AND FUNNELLED, SELF PROPELLING SHOPPERS. READY WITH CASH. HUGE TROLLEYS FOR GOODS. MASSAGE NOW OFFERED IN MALLS WITH HAIR AND NAIL CARE.

Transcendental Humming - Taking the Path Less Travelled

Wilma had moved to a new town, a very circular sort of place, a small rural hub, with two supermarkets and a Mall. It's religious and mining history uncomfortably lurched beside modern atheism, giving a dark and thoroughly unholy past and murky present to Wilma's eye. She and her husband had moved for work, the work had been there for him and plenty of it up to 12 hours a day, but the promise of a job for Wilma had not materialised and so she was playing a waiting game. To begin with, Wilma had joined a gym, getting up early to train with her husband and was using some of her day to valet for him, organising, unpacking and sorting their belongings. But as the days, weeks, months went by, the shadows of that place got longer, the days colder and Wilma felt the loss of her husband's comforting presence more and more, not the least because they had worked together for the past 25 years! Wilma started to walk to the mall, to fill in the gaps of self during the day. The colours of the "Get Stuffed" shop began to mesmerise her. She would stand in front of the blue and purple section in the thrall of the multiple shades; they beckoned to her, but then, she thought, what about the browns and pinks. Temptation lured her to begin trying things on, then to trying other things on. The mounting obsessional anguish of decisions laced with her brain chemicals racing about engaging the act to buy that thing! Wilma walked home with her presents, her emptiness assuaged for a few hours only. The next day the black holes would reappear and she would be right back at "Get stuffed" buying the next soul filler. The clothing heap was mounting up but the internal holes were getting bigger and bigger.

In the earlier chapters of this book we looked at the beginnings of a life, that of the developing child held within the caregiver's love. The caregiver has a "capacity for concern" which holds the child safely and which over time, the child internalises so that, it too can offer a capacity for concern towards itself, others and eventually, perhaps, its own children. Generally speaking, in the commercial world, the only capacity for concern relates to the financial rewards the companies, and their shareholders invest in. These, unfortunately for us, are the highway robbers who ride upon their dark rationalisations that it is the consumer's choice to eat or drink their product. When this product is dressed up, for instance as a health food, the subterfuge is that they are helping provide our nutritional choice's and adding to our perfection. The real entrapment of the consumer can be when the magic act of placing the dark and secret cloak over the "ingestible" happens; this is the mystical "rabbit in the hat" act. Food, as we know it, can be transformed through this magic act to be wrapped in colours, emanating amazing aromas, surrounded by food related sounds, tasting terrific and mouthwatering and, oh, the feeling of it...and this magic transformation act belongs in the realms of the unacknowledged, the very fine or invisible print. This act has changed the shape of the original food from the proteins, sugars and fats, the flour that it began life as and it has been transformed into another magical treat. If you have ever cooked anything, you will understand the alchemy of foods and the capacity we have to combine them and create a new entirely different object almost magically. By doing this our object constancy is overcome by alchemy.

It is the easiest game in town to pretend that anyone providing food products is trustworthy and honest, the tricks they can play with labelling are legend and there are many examples of mislabeling of products; Government standards and regulating teams spend their lives scouring their world attempting to catch those flouting the law or making new or updated laws in an attempt to capture new chemicals and new alchemic processes always trying to be outside the old regulations. Pick an ingredient, particularly additives, and try to decide what the number for that means. Without the "dictionary of definitions" and the eternal energy to look everything up, you're lost. Even if you can read the small print or invisible ink, it is an exhausting journey for the person who wants to know exactly what is in the food they are using for fuel and health for their wholistic future. Sad to say, it comes down to buyer beware, arm yourself with good defenses for the commercial capacity for concern is only for itself.

Developing a Taste for Water

They say that all life on this planet came from the sea, and the composition of people is 90%

water! However, growing up a long way from town water, farmers were reliant upon tank water and we often found the occasional dead bird floating in our drinking water! In the service of avoiding stomach bugs, the children were given boiled water combined with an orange liquid called 'quench' mixed with sugar to drink. No one drank water from the tap in case and so the water was used for teeth brushing, bathing, and boiling vegetables to death in.

When we lived in parts of SE Asia, drinking water became a commodity only found in those enormous bottles that were paid for and mounted on a filter and only the foolhardy risked brushing their teeth in the tap water! In the endless heat, water became priceless as dehydration is a major health hazard which is never to be taken lightly upon pain of passing out or severe headaches.

Consider for a moment, if you will, the huge amount of liquids sold as drinks. Now consider a caring owner of a real horse. Do you think, for a second, that they would think to give their horse anything to drink other than pure water?

It's the first choice of every living thing on the planet!

If it's not adding to your holistic life, then it's taking away!

Take Aways

Takeaways have become the great Take Away of Health. When it comes to nutrition it seems that takeaways have become a major contributor to the taking away of quality food choices. They have become a life preserver for the time-starved worker; we've all been there and done that, had takeaways because it is easier and everyone likes it. Fat and sugar are the cheapest and most addictive substances the commercial world can produce for us to ingest in large quantities.

The takeaways in the food industry are readily available and we don't have to think about what is in them, we trust the advertising: it says food. The ingredients in most takeaway foods are not written on the side of the wrapping. Here we are again in the realms of the Fantasy that it just disappears inside of us, and that it tastes so good makes us feel so good and so then we accept its disappearance. It's "fact" of being is discarded by the body and the mind in just the same way as the magical object disappears in the act. It's actually a take-away that adds!

The disappearing act of Food is incredible and unless we teach ourselves about the nature of food, the reality of food and the object constancy of food then we are doomed to never reach the Centaur of ourselves as our Horse and Rider have been cleft apart by the equation of food as fuel which is operated more and more by commercial operators.

If we can educate ourselves even slightly then the equation becomes an addition to the quality of our lives and not the undermining and thoroughly addictive takeaway process that it has become.

Without regular feeding with a minimum quality food our physiology is drained of the nutrients and subsequent energy it needs to function without becoming tired and blood sugar deficits occur. However our psychological state is often in denial of these physical needs as it has its own mission that has to be completed. If the Rider has obsessional plans and doesn't take into account the fact that their Horse is running on empty there's going to be a major breakdown! It's interesting to note going back to our motorist on their journey example from above, that most drivers operating a reasonable car would pick petrol for their car that has the best quality rather than just putting in the cheapest because it is convenient which is an interesting choice for performance from that engine don't you think?

So we have Quality

There are a lot of great foods that are available, easy to prepare and easy to transport anywhere on any journey. Taking supplies means organising resources for the integration of self, just like taking extra water for the car on a long journey, no one is there to fix your car for you in the desert: you are on your own if you break down!

It is a matter of training the Horse and Rider to eat together and not apart!

Understanding the constancy of food coming into being matters. This material world is one of a constant change of one type of material energy into another. Imagine this analogy: if all the food we ate just flowed straight out of us again, just as the overflow of petrol did, how would you have combustion for the engine to get anywhere?

So we have Constancy

We send a child to school with a certain amount of food, not three birthday cakes per day. So we think for the child's health.

The physical body does need a certain amount of protein per day to function well. If we can understand this from the psychological perspective as well as understand why we are eating or drinking what we do, keeping well becomes a much easier practice.

So we have Quantity

Getting an appraisal of how much fuel your individual psychophysiology requires can really help you decide what will work for your best energy levels.

The Equation of Centauring Regarding Food

First nature developing a conscious awareness and understanding using the Hindsight of our food habits: the why, when, and what Foods we eat, not just relying on Take-aways.

Insight: what is in the makeup of the food that we are integrating as a part of ourselves? This leads to the development of choices harnessing and harvesting the best positive energy from foods.

Foresight: how to plan for our energy output each day without making the load a burden.

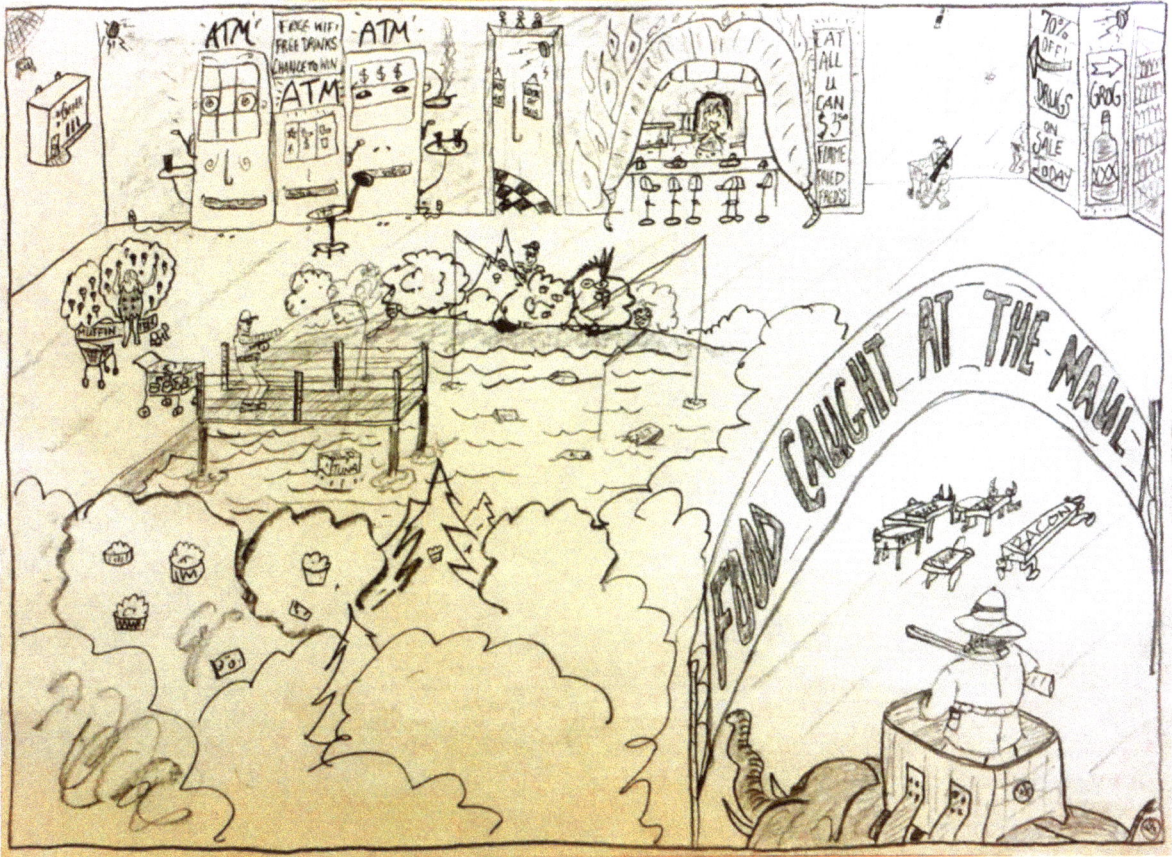

To that end, being able to eat small meals at regular intervals throughout the day, rather than the prescribed three meals actually helps your body metabolise the food more efficiently.

The chemical makeup of food is becoming more complex and the best key to understanding what you are becoming as you eat food is by using your higher defence mechanisms; become your own teacher, it's never too late to learn new tricks.

Denial, minimisation and rationalisations are still not good defenses for a Holistic health plan. The actual amounts of any kind of food do count when it comes to calories as they are the fuel we need for activity.

Some of the more interesting quotes, I have heard from the herd:

I only have a junk food day once a week

Everything I eat is healthy, I'm just a big eater

I don't like breakfast, so I don't bother

I don't have time to cook anything

I'm too lazy to be bothered, I'll just pick something up

They wouldn't sell it if it wasn't good for you

This is not a Takeaway, it's an Addition

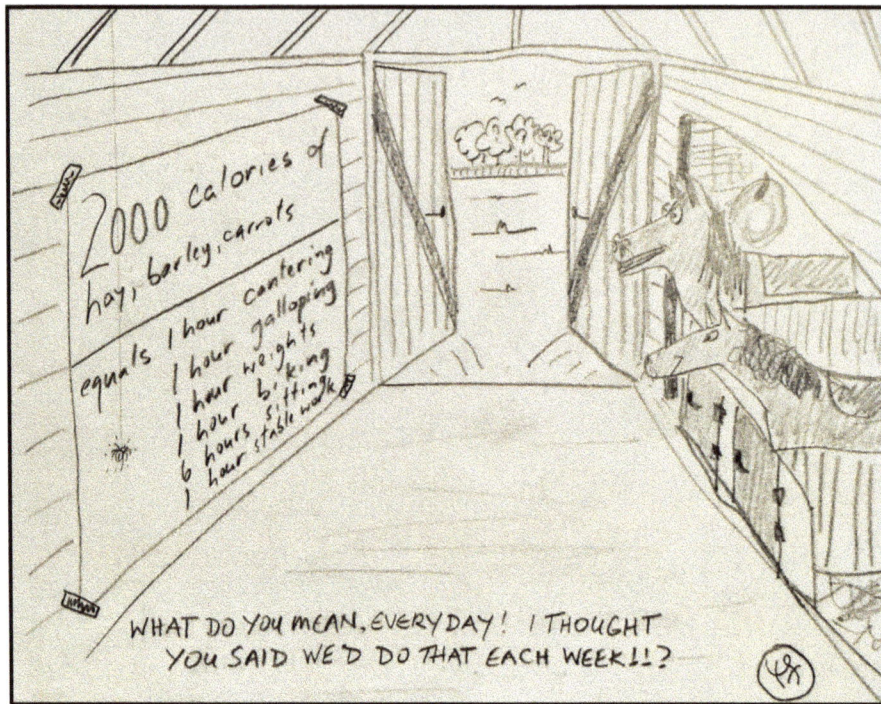

Start by being honest about what you eat and how much you eat. Apparently people are under reporting their calorie intake by half!

Yes, lean chicken breast is a very healthy meat, but a kilogram of chicken at one sitting is still going to have object constancy around your waist line even if you are running a marathon or a competing body builder.

When you undertake this part of the journey towards eating for your Centaur the best way to think about it is that the journey is about hunting and gathering the best foods for you and then deciding when and how much to eat of them for your best energy outputs and psychophysiology.

Craving foods essentially made of sugar, salt and fat, or what I like to call the ingestibles, as they have little to no nutritional value in them, even though they are taken orally; can feel overwhelming because we have evolved to hunt and gather these foods for survival. Famines were a part of the human experience well before the dawn of commercial foods. This meant that foods rich in fat or naturally occurring sugars were difficult to come by and we didn't have them as a common part of our diets. Our survival depended upon finding food or growing it ourselves and the search for it brought about an intrinsic fitness and psychological satisfaction, like the game of hide and seek. When we found fruit, nuts, seeds and meat, brain chemicals called endorphins were released into our being reinforcing the psychophysiological bond of this activity.

Thus it follows that we have an evolutionary anxiety built into our being of the fear of shortage of food. Our defenses are constructed to make sure eating is a first priority, remember that you were eating before breathing air, and so it follows that the discomfort from fear of famine is severe. Our brain chemicals are designed to signal hunger however if we train ourselves to eat small amounts of quality foods more often then these cravings will stop.

In the last century the Western world mechanised the global food industry and after the 1950's, in the Western world, there were no food shortages. If you look around the world now, it is impossible to find the famine in our society and stunningly, as of this year there are now more obese people in the world than underweight!

Remarkably, however, this is leading to a boom in malnutrition!

In what seems to be an unbelievably radical ironic twist, this is occurring in an epoch when there is more available food in the world than at any time in our history!

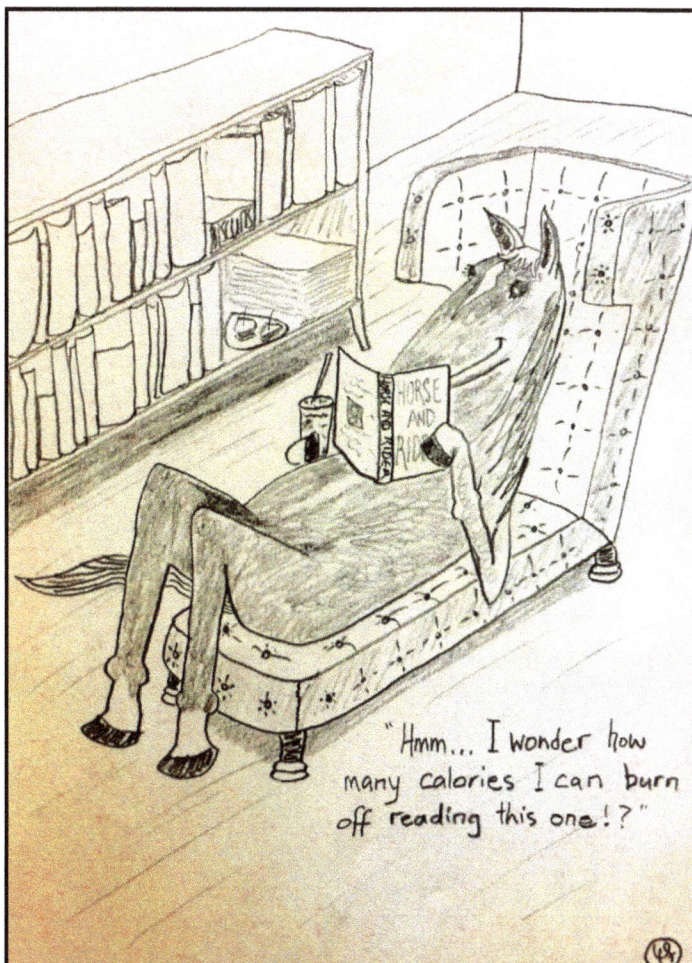

"Hmm... I wonder how many calories I can burn off reading this one!?"

By choosing the best quality foods rather than a larger quantity of poorer quality foods you will never be hungry again as you are giving your Horse and Rider exactly what they need. It is the same as when the infant cries and is fed in small shifts each day or night; you do not give it 3 bottles at a time, rather only one and then the next feed is some 4 hours later.

We do not have to eat just three times a day. This has been regulated over hundreds of years by our evolving society more to comply with the ever increasing demands of a work system developed to comply with the needs of productivity and profit naturally driven by commercial interests. It has nothing to do with healthy holistic eating for our psychophysiological system, we do much better not waiting until we feel starving hungry and then go searching for the quickest fix we can find which, these days will predictably be sugar, fat and salt.

How much do we need each day to satisfy the psychophysiological system?

Barbeques are a picnic; food to go; an art form of eating. They require of us to be planning ahead of the body. It is interesting to wonder about the magic of a barbeque and how gathering

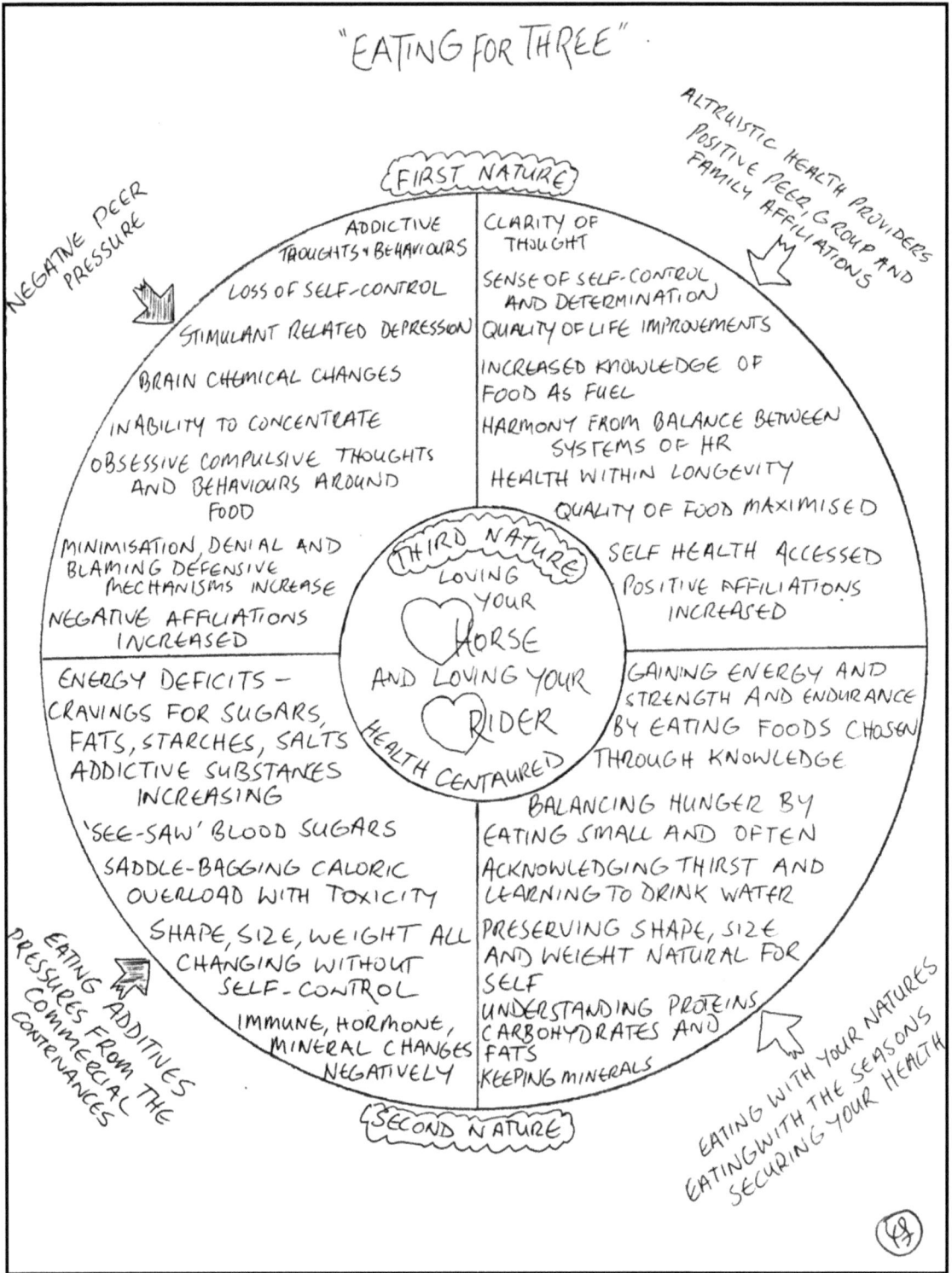

"EATING FOR THREE"

ALTRUISTIC HEALTH PROVIDERS
POSITIVE PEER, GROUP AND
FAMILY AFFILIATIONS

NEGATIVE PEER PRESSURE

FIRST NATURE

ADDICTIVE THOUGHTS & BEHAVIOURS

CLARITY OF THOUGHT

LOSS OF SELF-CONTROL

SENSE OF SELF-CONTROL AND DETERMINATION

STIMULANT RELATED DEPRESSION

QUALITY OF LIFE IMPROVEMENTS

BRAIN CHEMICAL CHANGES

INCREASED KNOWLEDGE OF FOOD AS FUEL

INABILITY TO CONCENTRATE

HARMONY FROM BALANCE BETWEEN SYSTEMS OF HR

OBSESSIVE COMPULSIVE THOUGHTS AND BEHAVIOURS AROUND FOOD

HEALTH WITHIN LONGEVITY

QUALITY OF FOOD MAXIMISED

MINIMISATION, DENIAL AND BLAMING DEFENSIVE MECHANISMS INCREASE

SELF HEALTH ACCESSED

NEGATIVE AFFILIATIONS INCREASED

POSITIVE AFFILIATIONS INCREASED

THIRD NATURE
LOVING YOUR ♥ HORSE
AND LOVING YOUR ♥ RIDER
HEALTH CENTAURED

ENERGY DEFICITS — CRAVINGS FOR SUGARS, FATS, STARCHES, SALTS ADDICTIVE SUBSTANCES INCREASING

GAINING ENERGY AND STRENGTH AND ENDURANCE BY EATING FOODS CHOSEN THROUGH KNOWLEDGE

'SEE-SAW' BLOOD SUGARS

BALANCING HUNGER BY EATING SMALL AND OFTEN

SADDLE-BAGGING CALORIC OVERLOAD WITH TOXICITY

ACKNOWLEDGING THIRST AND LEARNING TO DRINK WATER

SHAPE, SIZE, WEIGHT ALL CHANGING WITHOUT SELF-CONTROL

PRESERVING SHAPE, SIZE AND WEIGHT NATURAL FOR SELF

IMMUNE, HORMONE, MINERAL CHANGES NEGATIVELY

UNDERSTANDING PROTEINS CARBOHYDRATES AND FATS KEEPING MINERALS

EATING ADDITIVES PRESSURES FROM THE COMMERCIAL CONTENANCES

EATING WITH YOUR NATURES
EATING WITH THE SEASONS
SECURING YOUR HEALTH

SECOND NATURE

supplies for these is a much relished past-time all over the World but especially perhaps, here in the Antipodes.

When we take small children out the caregivers take bags of supplies: bottles pre-prepared with liquid food, nappies, teething rings, suntan lotion, squeaky toys and mashed up food. They really plan ahead for the child's psychophysiological needs.

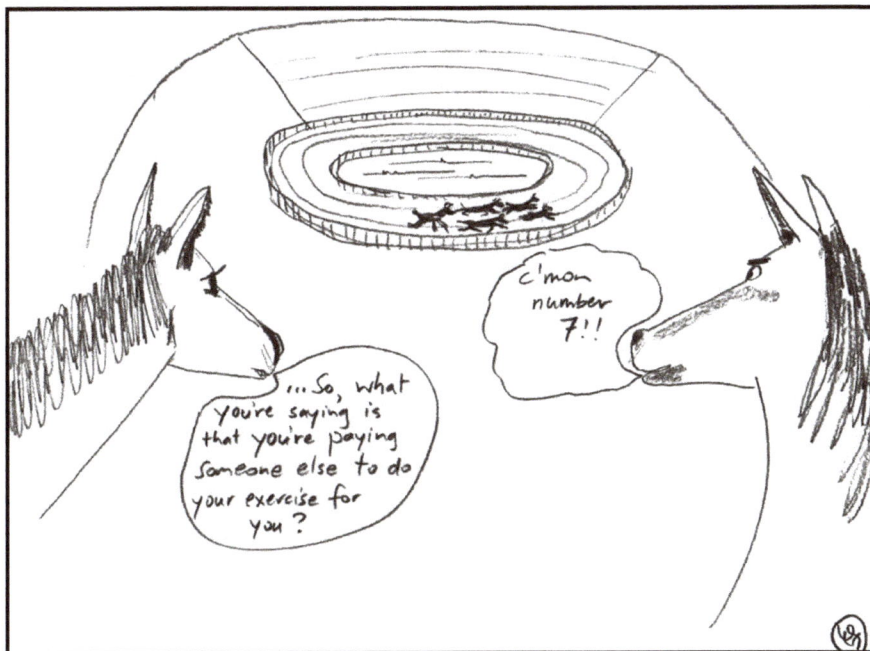

Quantity and Quality of Life

Ask yourself three questions:
1. How long do you want to live for roughly, just a ballpark estimate. A lot of us pick forever, right?
2. What kind of life quality do you want? In other words, what type of health? Would illness be part of this equation? How would you like your psychophysiological system to work for you?
3. Have you got any Active plan for Health in place apart from your GP, Dentist and life insurance?

A funny thing about planning and travel is, when you get on the plane they have a safety plan, you are told to put the oxygen mask over your own nose and mouth first, before trying to assist others, this is an imperative for your health survival plan! Statistics show those attempting to help even infants put on their oxygen masks first before putting their own on, pass out themselves due to lack of available oxygen. The point is to actively, consciously plan and then follow your plan for yourself. It is an imperative ingredient for discovering your Centaur and without it the journey becomes much, much harder.

Quote: *"You can't out exercise a Bad Diet!"*

Our psychophysiological being has a unique counting system developed eons ago to keep us alive and this inner calculator always knows deficit and surfeit. This system is on an automatic setting forever weighing up the equation of energy in, versus energy out. Everything going in counts and if more energy goes in than is needed, survival dictates that it be stored because of the long evolved anxiety of famine, but in the western world, as we have seen, we don't have famine we only have feasts. Long ago we hunted and gathered, walking, running and travelling from place to place for the foods we knew to be there. The food was rationed to fulfil energy out needs; no one sat in a car, or at a desk, or in front of a screen. Food gathering for our survival was our day time job, just as it is for every other life-form. The hierarchy of needs that we talked about in Chapter 1 which included those of shelter, food and water, clothing and foraging amongst other needs, took up all our time and energy. While we obviously still have needs, the energy output equation has radically changed and yet we are still burdened by our long evolved habits in relation to our eating.

Let's then look to actively lighten our load and unburden some of our saddlebags and by doing this we will take a load off our HR.

Pictures paint a thousand words so one of the most interesting exercises has us joining Horse with Rider and coming up with a very different mirror image than the one we are used to seeing. Mirrors can make huge psychophysiological differences, take for example:

The Mirror of the Photo Lens

Taking a photo of yourself standing in a relaxed pose can really help integrate the picture you have of yourself in your mind and the actual physical "you" that others see. Our defence mechanisms do sometimes make it difficult to register reality, as we have discussed in previous chapters. Taking a photo gives a starting point for the journey of holistic centauring as it gives you a real life baseline comparison of what your Horse looks like now to what kind of measurable outcomes you attain with your plan of action.

Stablemasters: Help is at Hand while Being Taken Care Of

Looking again at the higher defence mechanisms, we can see that once you have decided upon which adventure or path to embark on, anxiety quite often enters our Centauring Circle and can threaten to undermine our plans to effect change. However, the environment provides us with many choices of support in the form of caregivers or as I am calling them Stablemasters.

Personal trainers, Yoga teachers, physiotherapists, psychologists, dietitians are among the many professionals we can turn to and then there are often friends and family as well.

Grooming Intrinsic Motivations

As you are making changes to your psychophysiology how about thinking about feedback that is constructive and which helps you attain your goals.

Networking

Having a range of different people to focus on our holistic health gives multiple pathways to choose from such as a good hairdresser.

Long Term Goals in Adversity

Longevity and Suffering

We have talked at length about ordinary and difficult psychophysiological adversities that HR encounters in previous chapters. However there are those of us who have had even more major life crises and have already endured experiences that asked and took a great deal from us systemically. I think most would agree that it would not be out of turn to say that the longer we are on this planet, the more likely that a major grief or trauma will touch your life. I am often asked by parents how to find the perfect solution to saving their child from pain and sadness, and my answer has always been the same: that there is no magic shield, even our defenses cannot prevent reality from happening, though they do try. Things change and no matter how hard we want to hang on to someone or something, it is life's nature to come and go.

Because we begin with learning that people and objects have a certain constancy, a certain reliability in our World, it is written into our conscious mind for our psychological survival, that the Caregiver comes back. We etch their name upon our hearts and minds the minute we begin to love and remember them and they, in turn become a part of who we are.

We also internalise the fact that our arms, legs and physicality itself is stable and reliable as well, that they don't just disappear under the covers when we climb into bed. They too, are in fact constant even as they change and grow bigger.

The first two circles of our existence, Horse and Rider, line up consistently in unison as we have seen. The saddlebags we carry contain the history of the messages we grew up with and our defenses are there to help with our survival with adversities and experiences. Our first defenses had to be external, beyond ourselves and they were our caregivers. These people were our original shields from adversity and they stood with their arms around us in a perfect circle, until we developed internal strategies of our own which then enabled us to individuate from them, go out into the World and form other circles of our own.

What happens when the reality of either circle does in fact change, when for instance there are:

Psychological Losses Physical Losses
Parent, spouse or child dies Loss of a limb
Divorce Paralysis or accident
Loss of career Menopause
Loss of home

The ability to understand and find acceptance in our changing Natures is difficult as we are very rooted in the first two for our survival in a very material world. However, consider for a moment the existence of Third Nature; given that the Egyptians did not manage to take their bodies or their vast collections of personal belongings to an after-life, otherwise the Cairo Museum would be a much smaller place, not to mention the British Museum!

What do we draw upon in times of change, loss and adversity? Money and food may make a difference, however as we grow older the energy of food is not as necessary as when we were our younger selves. As of yet I don't think money has bought anyone immortality, only in the sense of what they left behind as memory or legend; see the pyramids again as a good example. So what is the reality of growing older in HR?

I believe that our Third Nature is there, right at our beginning, when the energy of love which accompanied all the physical and psychological care that our Caregivers gave us was given. Remember in Bowlby's research he found that it was not enough just to feed a baby, change its nappies and even to just hold it? The real difference to the child's ability to thrive came when the nurse actively began "loving activity" with the child. So love itself becomes the creative energy of Third Nature; we do things that we love to do, love is a verb, a doing word and an activity. It is also one of our greatest assets for Centauring.

The only energy source we have which can grow larger and larger over our lifetimes is our Third Nature or unconditional loving capacity. Some people develop this all of their lives, however it is an ever changing part of who we are and it is often developed from dealing with extreme adversity.

Quote - Every day in every way we are getting better and better!

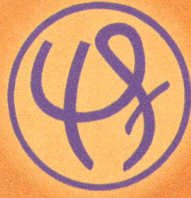

CHAPTER 5

PLANNING A HEAD FOR THE BODY,
OR A BODY FOR THE HEAD

'This world of ours, the world of Horse and Rider,
Was not conquered by the car,
Not conquered by the train,
Not conquered by plane,
But conquered bipedally'

Sara Beaumont-Connop

Now that we have both Horse and Rider eating together, we're ready to revisit some of our earlier themes which we introduced in Chapter 2 and 3. If you have followed the arguments presented so far you will know that movement is not really an optional arrangement if one wants to be a fully functional and Centaured being!

The "great drain" of inactivity leads to disharmony between our psychological and physiological dimensions; between our Horse and Rider. As we have seen, if anything splits our duality and separates Horse from Rider, it throws us from the saddle, and we cannot Centaur. This chapter is about changing the negative kinetics which prevent harmony of HR, into a positive energy flow, pictured a little like the "figure eight, infinity symbol", which then facilitates HR to enter the province of Centauring.

What is often apparent in the world today unfortunately, is that when the word "exercise" is mentioned a lot of negative connotations follow it immediately. It would be great to change "exercise", which is a word that can also mean writing in a school book, to an equivalent word like: having Fun and enjoyment of movement! That is really all it is; an extension of childhood activities we all loved to do like riding a bike, running, skipping, swinging, swimming, our whole bodies sang with the sounds of our movements. The other day I walked past a playground with swings and climbing frames and there were four goofy 20 year old young men playing together on the kiddy swings, you could see that they were transported back 15 or so years into their past and yet they were still in the present of being 5 years old again, having fun with movement!

We are of course, really discussing here the concept of Play which is something no ordinary child turns down the opportunity to engage with, for if it is an enjoyable act that they can derive pleasure from then they are going to plunge into it! This is of course dependent upon each individual as to what kind of play or exercise they may want to try.

Why would you want to choose to play with movement you may ask? Because we are de-signed to do it, as is every living thing. You have actually been doing it all your life! Can you remember when you slowed down and play changed to more sedentary activities such as watching TV or movies, or just surfing the Net, shopping or cruising around? There has been a flurry of research in recent years about the problems with just sitting down for hours at a time and the incredibly negative consequences this has on our psychophysiological patterns.

Quote: *"Idea's by themselves, cannot produce change of being; your effort must go in the right direction, and it must correspond to the other." P.D Ouspensky G.I Gurdjieff*

After spending a great deal of time watching children play and developing my own play routines for adults, I have developed a fundamental belief in the ability of playful exercise as a way of Centauring the self and preserving not only good mental health, but also good physical health which in turn is preserving psychophysicality longer and not only do Horse and Rider feel better for it but their functional interactivity increases rather than decreases as they get older; they Centaur themselves rather than the opposite!

Identification with Others: the Good, the Bad and the Ugly!

Quote: "Mirror mirror on the wall, who is the fairest of them all?"

This is a line from the well-known fairy tale Snow White. It is an archetype of the inbuilt psychophysiological survival mechanism we have evolved: the intrinsic need "to have whatever the neighbours have got, or to have one better!" We evaluate our environment all the time and measure ourselves up against all comers. Now, with social media having such a great impact on our psychology, advertisers marketing anything are able to manipulate this inbuilt desire to be perfect, using for instance, digital enhancements that are far beyond what we have been so far exposed to in the photographic world! In a parallel process to this, the medical cosmetic surgery industry has surged ahead with all manner of implants, uplifts, extensions, lasers, and fillers which lead us to an interesting juxtaposition that the psychology of the brain has been studied in order to capture the pleasure centres attention and to then exploit the concerns we have for our self-images. Both the commercial and medical world are advertising interventions for our various physical needs for "improvements" as something we can buy to augment perfection. These are marketed as a "cure" for anything including "ageing" and fears about the fact that we will die and not live forever.

As Doris made her way into the "mixed gym", she stood back in the main door way, "boy" it was busy! An aerobics class had just finished and a lot of slim, toned and beautiful young women streamed out of the far corner and into the weights room. All the men working out, stopped to stare. Doris felt her confidence withering and thought "Oh my God, what am I even doing here, everyone looks better that me, taller, slimmer, prettier; even the guys, how can I compete with all those women? I don't have streaming blonde hair or a butt that is that good!" She felt the fear, she felt the anxiety and the envy, but she also felt another part of herself saying, "Ok, so you are not a gazelle, you will never be a gazelle, because you are an ocelot; no one else is you and they can never be you with your eyes, your exact physicality, your smile or who you are, and you might even make some good friends out of some of them too!"

Will you spend your life wishing you were someone else, when you won the right to be you, the only you that there ever has been or will ever be? Doris turned to the mirror, switched on her best smile and walked into the room.

Finding a role model is useful and smart, if it empowers us to "be the best individual, we can be!" Living your life and trying to capture the elusive shadow of another's psychophysiology could be the greatest futility and loss that one could sustain, to be anyone but yourself depletes this world of your uniqueness!

How do we avoid the traps and snares of feeling inferior? This is when a mentor, partner or friend who values and understands your individual needs is most helpful and can guide and support you through self-doubt and fear of failure. This allows a screen to block out others and a focus on the play. Remember the first day at school or a new job? If at school then you were met by the teacher or at work, a supervisor. You were given a desk and introduced to peers, you were helped to understand what was expected of you with the work tasks. Most of us did not just turn up and know how to cope with all the new experiences by ourselves. New experiences take time to learn and we need help to learn and adapt to new surroundings and tasks. We ask for help at work and at school and this is the same principle we use now.

Reflections on Who we are and How we are: Mirrors and making the most out of our psychophysiology.

As outlined earlier in the book, our parents are our first mirror of movement, we watch and imitate them, extending ourselves into space. If we have them, siblings or other children are next, our appetites for emulation are voracious and we are forever questing for new combinations and tricks, swinging, climbing, jumping come next, teaching us invaluable lessons about our Horse.

Without these first Mirrors we would not have as much information about how our physicality works. It is a natural part of human development to copy what others do. Following this learning, we move up to the transference of the mirroring task to a more abstract concept. This is the ability to be alone with the "parent mirror" in our mind's eye and to translate what we have observed watching them and practice it in an actual mirror checking our movements or looking at the way we appear and stand. Everyone as a child, who grew up with a mirror somewhere in their house, found their way to the magical glass and practiced faces, poses or if they were lucky, and the mirror had "wing mirrors", looked into the fantastical infinity of self they could make by pulling the wings to look at each other! Now, when we go to a gym, a dance studio or we learn from a yoga teacher we will always find either that we are mirroring the teacher or that our movements are mirrored back to us by mirrors of some kind reflecting our postures in movement.

Working in a gym for years was an incredible opportunity on so many levels. On day one, the first thing I had to get used to were the Mirrors, they were everywhere, on every wall. I would on occasion look up and suddenly catch a reflection of my body hunched over at the shoulders as I rounded forwards. My first experience of "catching" myself leaning towards kyphosis, which was not great! I had never noticed that before; here

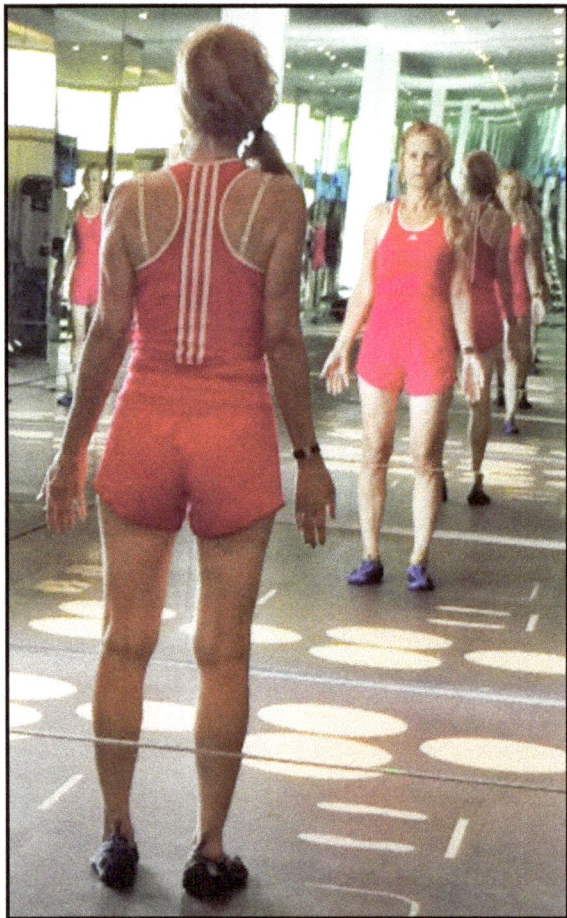

To Infinity and Beyond

I was, doing every exercise in the gym trying to earn a great physique and my posture was letting me down. I started to practice every time I caught my mirror image by standing up tall, shoulders back and down and I found that by pulling my chest and back up, that this in turn led to my lungs filling with oxygen more freely! This in turn meant that I was breathing better, standing taller and remarkably, it also made my stomach flatter and my muscles tighter. This was an incredible discovery and it is one of the most simple yet fundamental elements we need to practice, consciously in the moment; as it facilitates Horse and Rider to move toward Centauring and balance so easily.

Body Language, the Horse is Talking Back, Literally!

Most of us are aware that when we are tired, our chest caves in and our shoulders hunch forward and down. This is just one of a number of movements the Horse uses to communicate its physical feelings holistically to the Rider; it is hopefully true, that the Rider is aware of the significance of this message! The holistic benefits of learning about one's posture are phenomenal as they allow us into the dimension of movement inhabited by our health and our Centaur. Most of us do not have perfect posture; we all have idiosyncratic ways of holding our physicality, luckily this can be assessed by a physiotherapist or a good personal trainer.

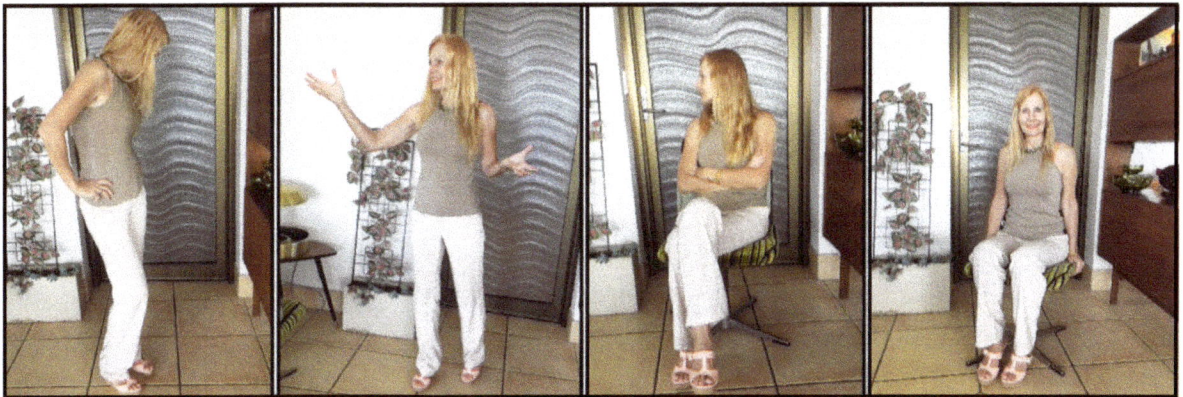

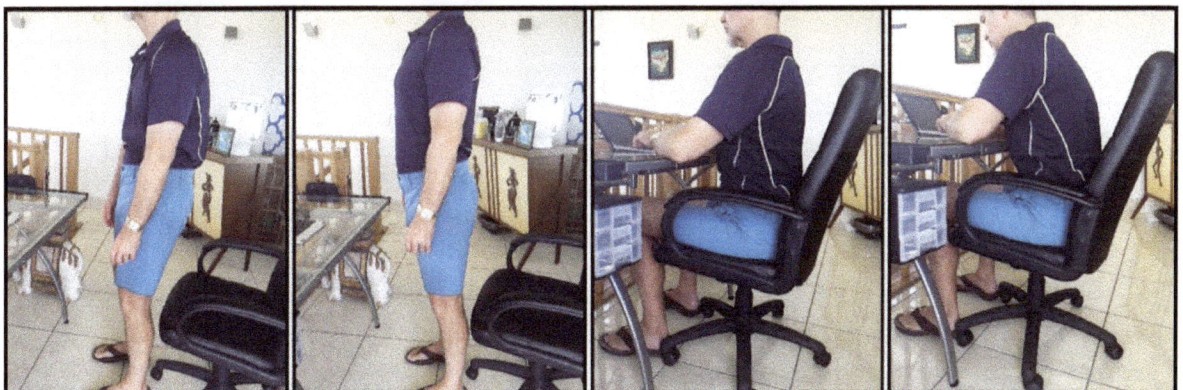

PSYCHOPHYSIOLOGY OF POSTURE

FIRST NATURE

NEGATIVE PSYCHOLOGICAL

Depression
Fearful and timid
Bored and tired
Anxious
Despairing
Powerless   Angry
Uptight   Dysfunctional

Exaltation
Confident
Ready   Motivated
Empowered
Peaceful   Alert
Functional
Relaxed

POSITIVE PSYCHOLOGICAL

"How You move IMPACTS ON How You FEEL"

Rounded shoulders
Hollow chested
Flat pelvis   Bent over
Limping
Twisted up   Weak
Crooked
Sitting Slumped

Standing tall
Energetic
Fascinated   Strong
Sexy
Alive   Vibrant
Turned on
Sitting erect

NEGATIVE PHYSICAL

POSITIVE PHYSICAL

SECOND NATURE

HOW YOU MOVE IMPACTS ON HOW YOU FEEL IMPACTS ON HOW YOU MOVE IMPACTS ON HOW YOU FEEL IMPACTS ON HOW...

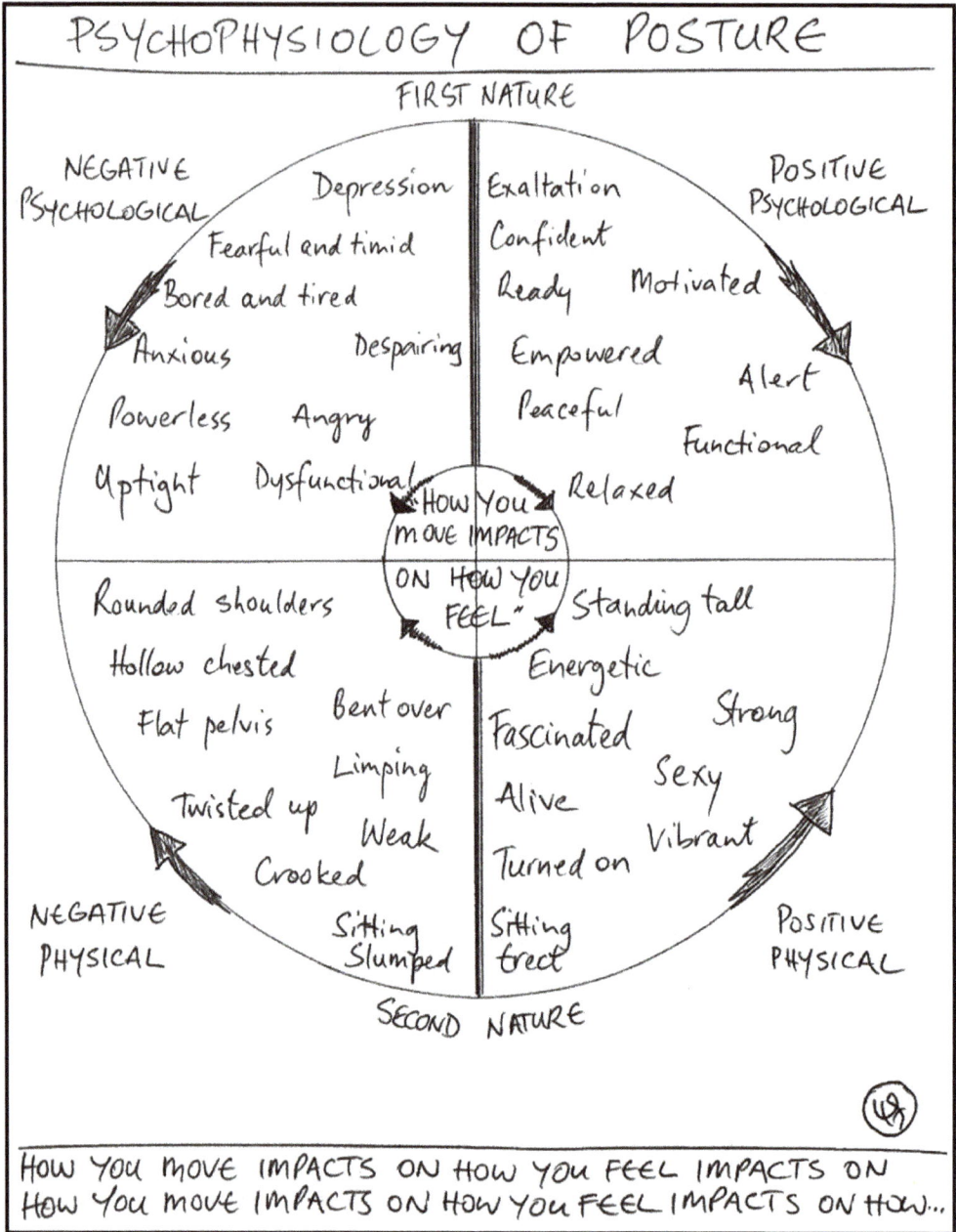

The Three Sights

Hindsight: What has happened to your body to create its aches and pains?
Insight: How has your body responded to these hurts by holding itself in certain positions?
Foresight: What you can do by stretching and developing your physique, with reference to

your posture, to assist you avoiding future injury and correcting your posture as much as possible. For example, stretches and exercises to correct lordosis.

Stretching the Mind to Stretch the Body

Because we don't see the bones we own, that is unless we have the misfortune of breaking one; they become part of the invisible object constancy we talked about in the previous chapters. In other words, we know they are there as they hold our body upright! We all have probably seen someone else's skeleton in pictures or hanging about in a classroom but usually these skeletons never have any of the muscles attached to them! The muscles themselves are the whole pulley and lever system of our physicality and so, not surprisingly, no one moves without them! Our muscles are indispensable and without them operating efficiently we are essentially sidelined. Keeping our Horse well by exercising and feeding it as lovingly as we can ensures HR system has the greatest chance in life.

The Oral Olympics: The First Activity of the Mind

As someone who has spent virtually my whole life talking, it occurred to me that speech is very symbolic of the different kinds of energies that have great impact upon our lives. From early conception we heard talking sounds, they brought us into the world and were some of the first symbols for our minds to make sense of. In fact, we are dependent upon this energy for our social survival. Try going to a country where you don't understand the language. Suddenly your ability to be an independent adult in the world who can get things done is severely reduced. Talking is the first step on the ladder to motivate the child to achieve its milestone movements and the harnessing of this energy can lead large crowds to do incredible things! Just attend a lively political rally or a concert; these have a magical creative energy and movement. Note that these examples are at the other end of the spectrum to the "help rejecting and complaining" defenses we were introduced to in Chapter 2, of which energies can only lead to dead ends.

Freud wrote about his talking cure as being the "Royal Road to the Unconscious", or, in his mind, the best way to discover our defence mechanisms. This is true in the sense that hidden or negative emotions can be released in cathartic ways. Releasing these disguised thoughts and feelings are healing for the client as they can facilitate understanding and therefore lead to changes in the individual's choice of more mature defenses. It interesting to note that Freud spend his lunch hour walking a route every day to a park near his home office in Vienna, whist thinking and constructing his theory. When I walked this same route some years ago, I began to think about the steps to take after the talking cure had been effected.

What about the physical movement towards the centaur?

I postulated the need to balance movement in both directions:

Seated: − − − − −   is the talking cure.

Standing: | | | | | is the walking cure.

And together equals the Wholistic cure: +

Taking baby steps made you the physicality you are today, or to put it another way Rome wasn't built in a day! That our body is going to grow from our child size to our adult size by itself essentially, is an implicit belief that we all have! It is another example of the object constancy thinking and understanding which is based on reality testing with others. Remember that it stands to reason we did not get to adulthood overnight, that one major meal did not get us from 1 year old to the 20 year old right?

Movement and exercise work in exactly the same way that food does: it is an incremental alchemy which the mind and body work with. We can only join up the dots slowly! So it is not remarkable that there are no overnight sporting successes; all physical feats are based on moments which have been practiced and repeated virtually every day, repetitively, and that includes just walking. The less you do a movement the less you can do it! Our fitness level goes up and down according to how often we do the movements and so does our weight and so do our thoughts about how we feel.

This constant duality is who we are and without the practice of joining HR together in thought and planning through to actions and movements including exercising and eating our duality becomes distant and unrelated and we are reduced to a kind of nothing. Exercise is making an investment in your holistic self; so how much are you worth? I believe your life makes you priceless, don't you? Wouldn't you rather invest in yourself instead of, for instance, the medical or insurance system, so that they get the boat, the new car, the overseas holiday and you are too sick to go?

I have found it interesting to see the daily routines, activities and exercises that people will adhere to without much fuss; mainly if they are going out to work or to a club:

Doing their Hair

Brushing their Teeth

Washing their face

Shaving

Applying face cream or cologne

Make up

Dressing carefully

Wearing their best jewellery

Eating

Remarkably, or not, the majority of the daily discipline of just about everybody is focused on the head, we spend 80% of our daily exercise focusing from our neck up! Our heads are almost the only pieces of ourselves that we are concerned about. How many people look in a full length mirror?

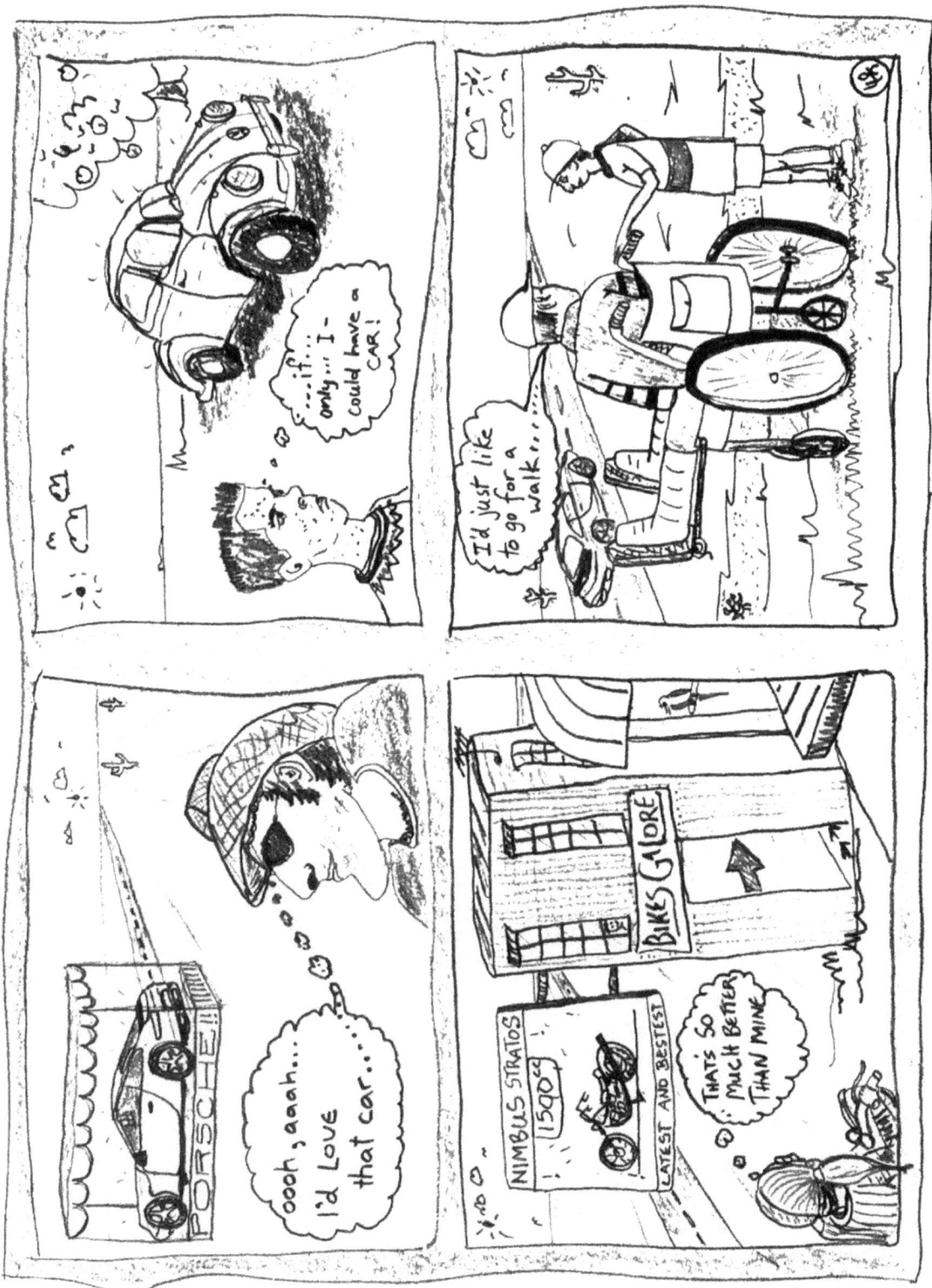

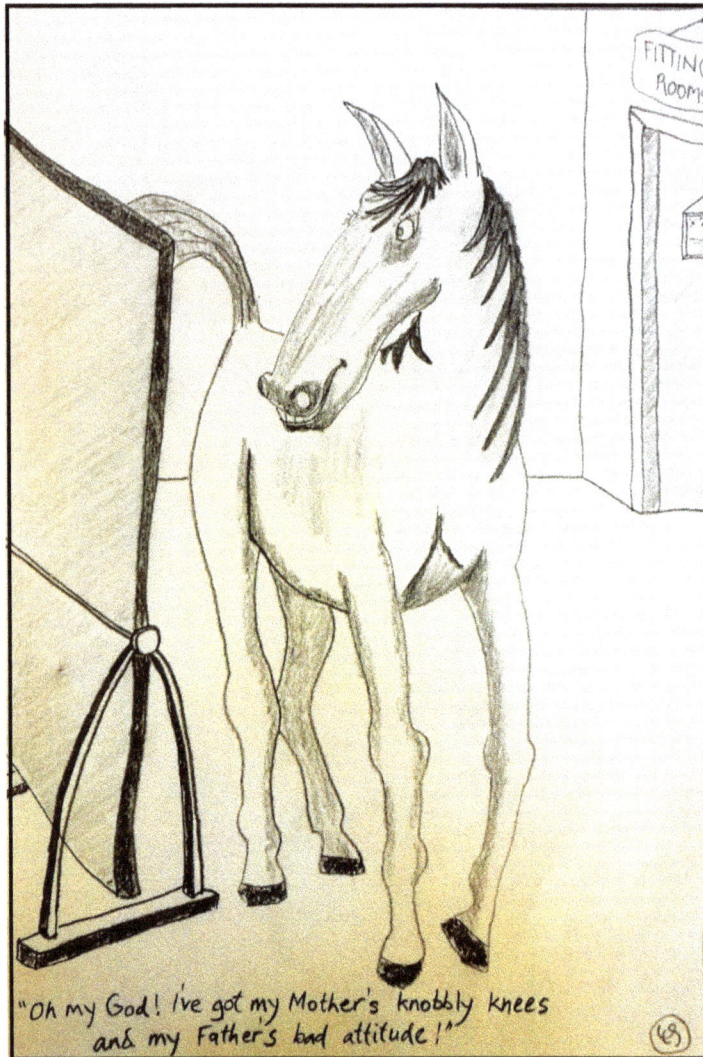

"Oh my God! I've got my Mother's knobbly knees and my Father's bad attitude!"

Taking Passionate Pathways

Whatever the movement we choose, I believe it has to contain elements of enjoyment, fun and harmony which when harnessed will build up to exertion and harmonic exertion is the goal. We have to go from external motivators to intrinsic motivators: To begin with just walking can be a first step, and yes, please excuse the pun. Understand and accept the fact of your duality. Begin to practice by opening up a conversation with yourself and talk with your Horse and imagine what you would enjoy playing! Do you remember something like this: At school the bell rings for lunch and the children have about 40 minutes after eating to play? The majority of them jump up and roar off to play a game; they just know what they are going to do or they are astute enough to choose an activity and someone to do it with really quickly in the 40 minute window of opportunity.

When they arrive back in class they are usually a much more relaxed and centaured group!

If you go back to Chapters 2 and 3 and remember how you have been using your défenses historically, you can begin to see how to harness them in the service of your physiology. Obviously you need to be able to think about these and perhaps discuss with a mentor or stable master what your blocks to movement are and how to use or develop your better defenses to re-Centuar yourself and move forward.

Whispering One's Self Hoarse

What about the Dark Horses or nightmares, the aspects of self which we will refer to as the silhouette of the self?

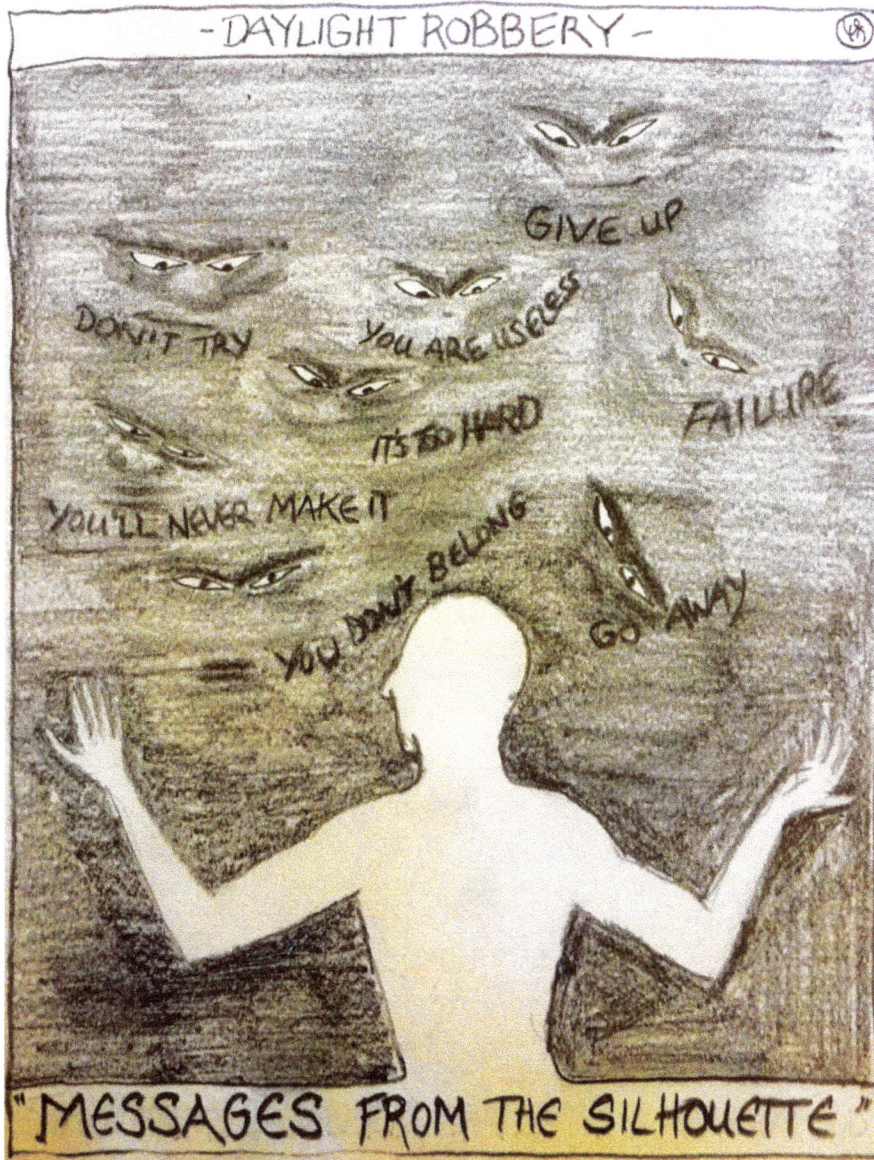

As we grow up, a lot of information from our external reality is projected on to every individual's physiology, these are the ideals of our society's norms. What we should wear, how we should move and look and these norms shape our internal library of images, which in the classified section come with their very own negatives. These are messages which accompany the negatives, so you can have a movie! Unfortunately they often show physical failures and public humiliations; our losses in competitions, failures which can defeat our mind and our body in quests to win. Often, when we are not Centaured, we replay these experiences in our minds eye because these are the hurdles that hurt the most! Just because physical pain has stopped, does not mean it is over and forgotten; most of us are not running back to the dentist unless it's a crisis moment!

These silhouettes are like highway robbers riding the black horses. They can accost us on our journey towards achieving our goals and success, they steal our will-power and energy by immersing us in a deluge of feelings and thoughts by calling out in unison "Give up, you can't do it, it's too hard, you don't have the time; go and watch TV, you already worked hard today. No one cares if you don't do it, it doesn't matter." These negative psychophysiological memory stories lurk about waiting. It is up to us to acknowledge them in the light of understanding, by using our hindsight to develop fresh insight and see how they rob us of confidence and commitment to be active in our self-care. Then, and only then, can we use our foresight to plan strategies and move towards a more Centaured self.

Preventing these thieves from dragging us off our paths and committing daylight robbery is a full-time job, for every day they are waiting to pull us down as we take each hurdle. They are internally represented as: stress, fatigue, self-doubt, boredom, pain, anger, disillusionment and they can appear to us externally as traffic jams, difficult relationships with others, long hours at work, accidents, bad coffee, money problems or more seriously loss, grief and depression.

These dark horses pillage our self-esteem as they threaten to drown the positive physical and psychological images we have fought to create. It can feel as though they are pulling us down until we join them in the black pools of our minds, lost and sunk into our younger defenses, those of denial, blame, minimisation and help rejecting complaining for instance. Our journey is split away from our goals, as we have been divided off from our Centaur. We then forget our purpose of dual, harmonious growth and focus only on "getting ahead"; in other words, of thinking only First Nature survival strategies. It is then that our Horse is veiled; we have lost sight of the whole picture and we have been reduced to just keeping our head above water, water which threatens to drown us.

Domestication of any animal takes away or at least tones down their wild nature. For example cats and dogs have become totally dependent upon their human caregiver for their entire lives. This includes what they are fed, when they are fed, how much they are fed; what happens when they are sick or injured, or how much space they are allowed and if they are given exercise opportunities or any play time.

Pearl's Story

Sometimes wild ideas can fly into one's head as they are trying to express that person's life at "full speed" and that is how it was for Fiona. She wanted to get a pet that would fulfil the fantasies that Bob, her husband had had as a child. These were of beautiful and colourful parrots who were all magical "squawkers and talkers" and who sat on shoulders and were delightful comedic companions. It was Bob's birthday coming up and Fiona scoured the pets for sale columns, and there it was, the advertisement which would bring fantasy to reality: Cockatoo's for sale. They journeyed to pick up their Pearl; she was pure snow-white with a sulphur crest and it was love at first sight as she immediately sat on Bob's shoulder all the way home and snuggled in a cloud of talcum scented feathers.

What about the human animal; are we domesticated by the external societal system that we live in?

Capitalism, while the currently indispensable, does contribute in no small part to this process, as we spend most of our daylight hours at a job which is now more often conducted in an office space where the greatest opportunities are provided for sitting down at desks on chairs and at meetings. It has become difficult for most people to get to go "outside" into a naturally beautiful world during a working day in order to go for a walk or to just stretch out our muscles. We are caged, in the sense that hourly breaks are not usually mandated nor are they usually tolerated. This work-life balance, or lack of balance is facilitated by a system that uses two of the most incredible motivational reinforcers, those of Money and Food.

Inpatient for Change and Growth

The biological imperative running throughout our entire lives is to develop, to grow and to change. Many adults however, remarkably have expectations that their physiology, will either stay the way it was when they were in their late teens, or that it will somehow magically change when they do something once or twice a week! It is interesting to note that an adult body took about 18 years to construct, moment by moment and minute by minute! All of these moments and minutes were made up of actions and movements, these then added up over those 18 years meant that you performed a lot of exercises just to get to eighteen, as we have previously discussed!

The greatest thing about being human in my opinion, is that it doesn't matter what you look like or how bad you may feel, there are things that you can change!

Physiology can be changed; your body itself has a health memory built right into it and it wants to be Centaured. All of the defenses our Rider uses can be understood and the saddlebags we have loaded up onto our Horse can be unloaded with care, time and patience. Just as the caregivers who facilitated your uniqueness and your beginnings assisted your growth into an independent adulthood with their belief, so too can you facilitate the changes you may want and need through your own efforts and beliefs. Even when things went wrong they helped make a plan for you to make changes for your holistic health and you accomplished them and so, if you are reading this book now, you have succeeded with a great deal of psychophysiological challenges already!

Taking a Breath Forward, giving yourself the "Kiss of Life"

It is interesting that the instant first aide for victims of drowning and for those who have stopped breathing, is to attempt to give breath. Oxygen masks are found in all emergency vehicles, but how often do we stop to consider and understand just how remarkable our own

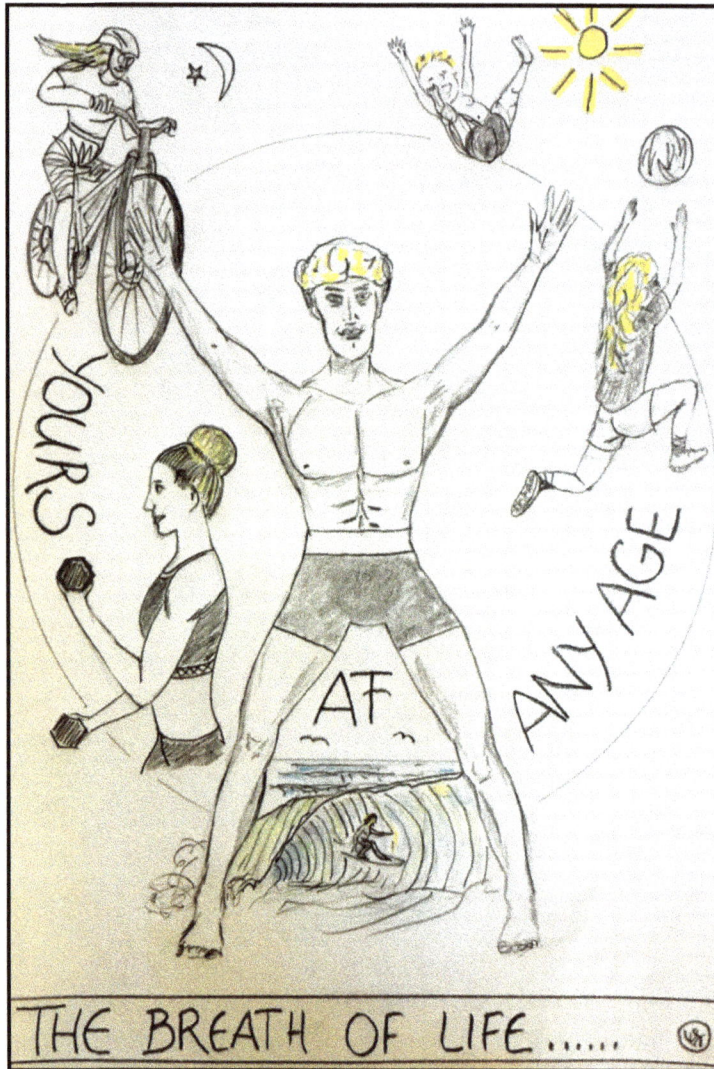

YOURS AT ANY AGE

THE BREATH OF LIFE......

breathing really is?

Taking a breath, which was the first thing we did when we entered the non-fluidic world, filled our lungs with air, and we could not have survived without it! The breaths we take, decide how much exertion we can perform, so if the oxygen supply is limited, so too is movement and at times the inability to breathe normally can lead to panic attacks which then limit any bodily functions effectively sidelining both Horse and Rider!

Just being able to take breaths that are healthful can help with endurance in any activity or stressful situation, the calming effect of doing the first exercise that you ever attempted gives energy to carry on with your endeavours. Oxygen enables our minds and our muscles to function in unison. Just try holding your breath when attempting to walk upstairs and see how far you get; then try the opposite exercise: take small breaths often and breathe your way up the stairs, you will find it a lot easier. We produce a harmony within our duality of psychophysiology when we harness our Natures in tandem. This harmony, which can lead to the feeling of being Centaured, is a beautiful, yet ephemeral thing, lasting for a finite time only. It is because it lasts for only a short time that many of us, who have not experienced it often, forget it. Being breathless is only useful in awe inspiring situations and even then you have to take a deep breath to take it all in.

The following exercise is possibly the most useful intervention assisting those suffering from anxiety and panic, once any danger has either passed or is being effectively dealt with.

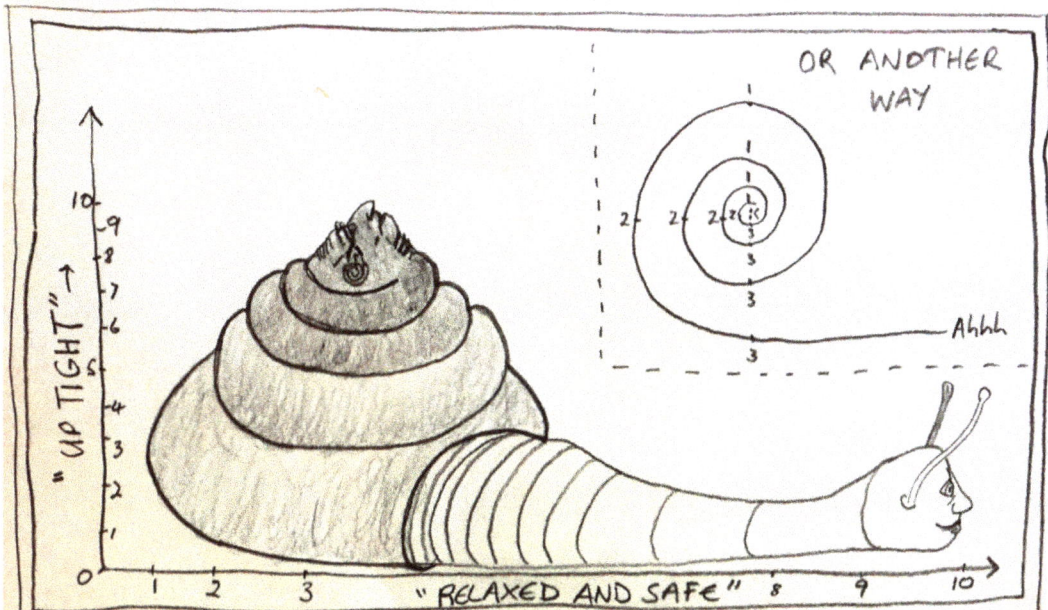

"TO THE "COUNT OF THREE"

Be somewhere quiet and safe, go walking if you can —
1. Breath in through your nose to the count of 3...
2. Once you are full, hold to the count of 3...
3. Breath out through your mouth, to the count of 3...
4. Once you are empty, hold to the count of 3...
5. Repeat 1-4 a lot

The count of 3 will be faster at the start,
because you are tight, may be with fright...

The count of 3 will slow down as you go,
because you've relaxed and gone with the flow...

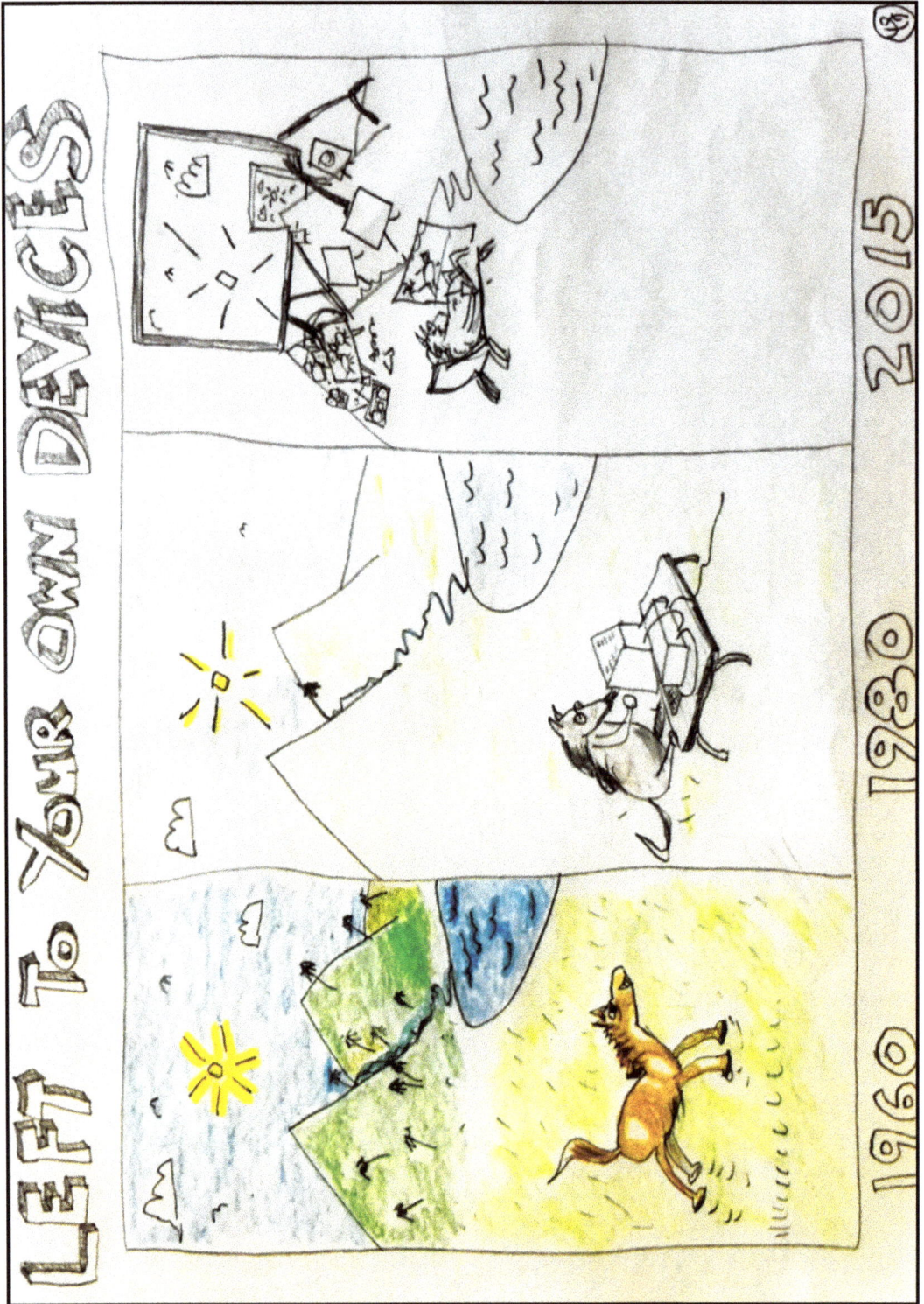

Here's a Playful Activity from the Stable Master of this Book

Take a 30 minute walk anywhere enjoyable, take a friend if you like, rehearse activities in your mind, how could you improve your psychophysiology?

What incentives and motivators can you come up with for yourself, your partner, family, friends?

A lot of people decide they want to join in with other people's games, such as joining groups already organised with a leader, like Yoga, gyms, boot camp, running groups, biking groups, aerobics for instance.

Why and How would using Exercise help with Adversity?

Seven years ago, my friend, Maryann, retired. She had been a special needs teacher her whole adult life, a caring and positive, hardworking and diligent woman with a passionate love of life and a tremendous desire to facilitate it for anyone who needed her help. After six months of her new life, she woke up one morning to an avalanche of stress. Her husband, also a teacher throughout his entire life, was diagnosed with bowel cancer and needed immediate surgery. For the next five years, this situation became a war, waged operation after operation; they sat on the brink of despair, never knowing what would go wrong next! Sitting in waiting rooms as her husband underwent procedure after procedure, Maryann's own psychophysiological system weakened naturally. After seeking a lot of psychological support, with much discussion focused on understanding her own traumatic state of being, she planned taking "waiting walks" outside in the grounds of the hospital while practicing rhythmical breathing. Finally the need for hospitalisations slowed down, but the visits to specialists continued unabated, as the next diagnosis given was Parkinson's disease; so now they faced a second battlefront and Maryann knew she would need a much bigger plan of attack for this one!

Let's look at Maryann's and Iain's defenses and their Centauring Circles:

Centauring Circle at Work

Long term goal strategies for Maryann and Iain:
Ability to deal with changing adversity over time.
Joining support groups to acknowledge the problems and issues with others input.
Getting a dog to help with having fun while walking everyday.
Physiotherapy to assist with the stiffening up of physiology.
Joining an art group to express emotion and maintain fine and gross motor movement.
Joining a ladies biking group for fitness and social opportunities.
Going to a gym to develop upper body strength and maintain bone density.
Downsizing the property for safety and health: less house and yard work.

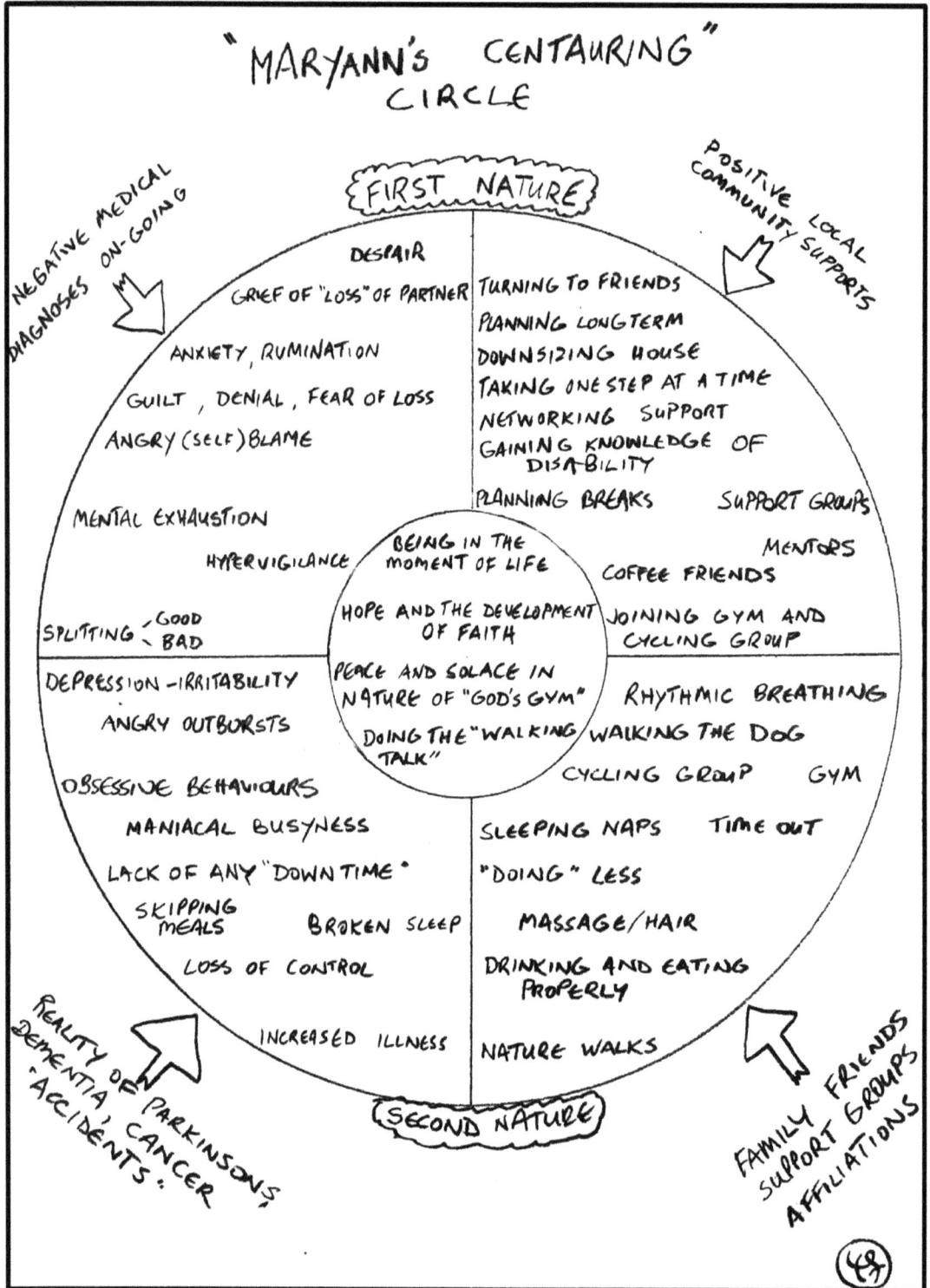

"MARYANN'S CENTAURING" CIRCLE

FIRST NATURE

NEGATIVE MEDICAL DIAGNOSES ON-GOING

POSITIVE LOCAL COMMUNITY SUPPORTS

DESPAIR
GRIEF OF "LOSS" OF PARTNER
ANXIETY, RUMINATION
GUILT, DENIAL, FEAR OF LOSS
ANGRY (SELF) BLAME

MENTAL EXHAUSTION
HYPERVIGILANCE
SPLITTING - GOOD / BAD
DEPRESSION - IRRITABILITY
ANGRY OUTBURSTS
OBSESSIVE BEHAVIOURS
MANIACAL BUSYNESS
LACK OF ANY "DOWN TIME"
SKIPPING MEALS   BROKEN SLEEP
LOSS OF CONTROL
INCREASED ILLNESS

TURNING TO FRIENDS
PLANNING LONGTERM
DOWNSIZING HOUSE
TAKING ONE STEP AT A TIME
NETWORKING SUPPORT
GAINING KNOWLEDGE OF DISABILITY
PLANNING BREAKS   SUPPORT GROUPS
MENTORS
COFFEE FRIENDS
JOINING GYM AND CYCLING GROUP
RHYTHMIC BREATHING
WALKING THE DOG
CYCLING GROUP   GYM
SLEEPING NAPS   TIME OUT
"DOING" LESS
MASSAGE/HAIR
DRINKING AND EATING PROPERLY
NATURE WALKS

BEING IN THE MOMENT OF LIFE
HOPE AND THE DEVELOPMENT OF FAITH
PEACE AND SOLACE IN NATURE OF "GOD'S GYM"
DOING THE "WALKING TALK"

SECOND NATURE

REALITY OF PARKINSON'S DEMENTIA, CANCER 'ACCIDENTS'.

FAMILY FRIENDS SUPPORT GROUPS AFFILIATIONS

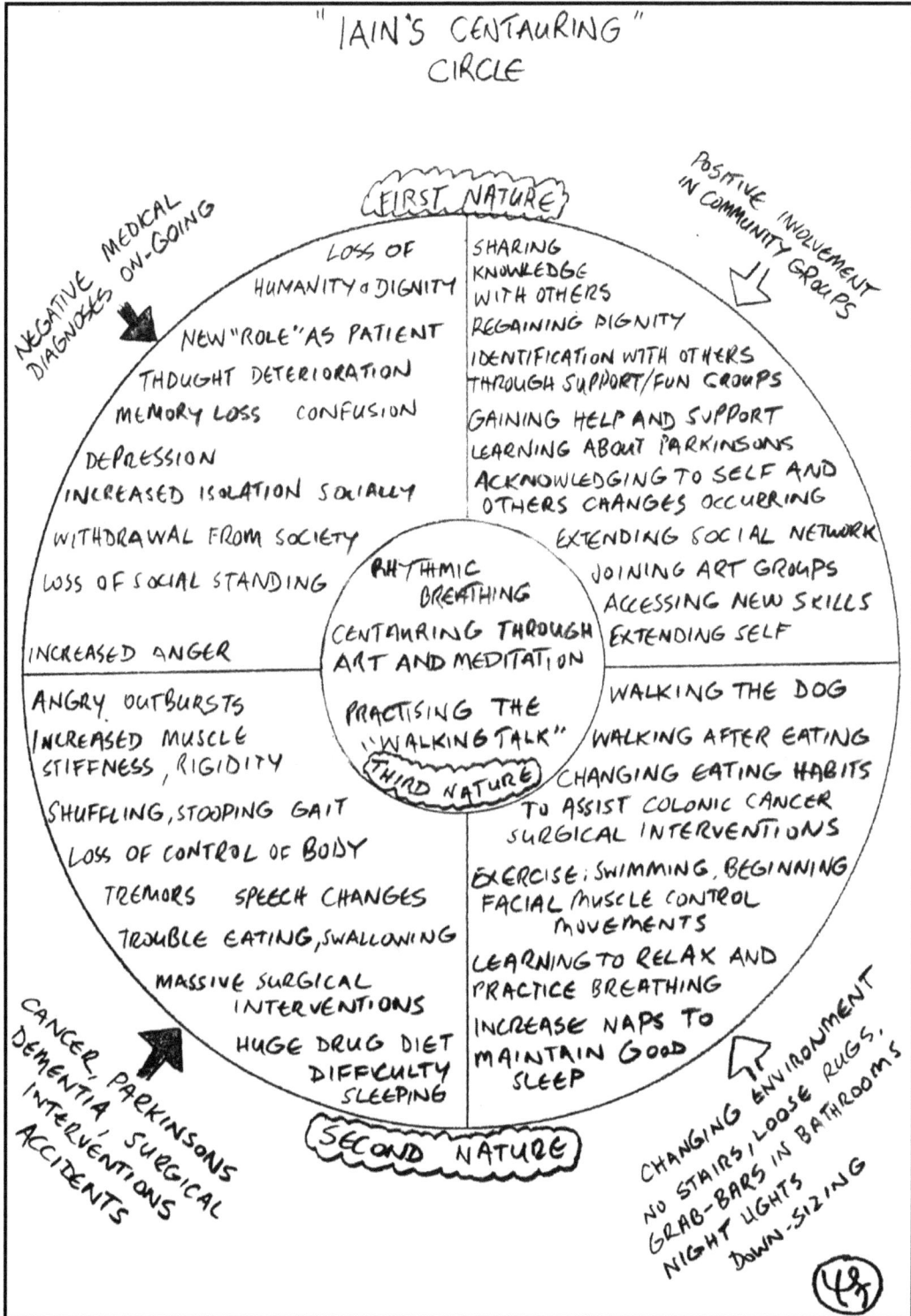

"IAIN'S CENTAURING"
CIRCLE

FIRST NATURE

NEGATIVE MEDICAL DIAGNOSES ON-GOING

POSITIVE INVOLVEMENT IN COMMUNITY GROUPS

LOSS OF HUMANITY & DIGNITY
NEW "ROLE" AS PATIENT
THOUGHT DETERIORATION
MEMORY LOSS   CONFUSION
DEPRESSION
INCREASED ISOLATION SOCIALLY
WITHDRAWAL FROM SOCIETY
LOSS OF SOCIAL STANDING

INCREASED ANGER

ANGRY OUTBURSTS
INCREASED MUSCLE STIFFNESS, RIGIDITY
SHUFFLING, STOOPING GAIT
LOSS OF CONTROL OF BODY
TREMORS   SPEECH CHANGES
TROUBLE EATING, SWALLOWING
MASSIVE SURGICAL INTERVENTIONS
HUGE DRUG DIET
DIFFICULTY SLEEPING

SHARING KNOWLEDGE WITH OTHERS
REGAINING DIGNITY
IDENTIFICATION WITH OTHERS THROUGH SUPPORT/FUN GROUPS
GAINING HELP AND SUPPORT
LEARNING ABOUT PARKINSONS
ACKNOWLEDGING TO SELF AND OTHERS CHANGES OCCURRING
EXTENDING SOCIAL NETWORK
JOINING ART GROUPS
ACCESSING NEW SKILLS
EXTENDING SELF

WALKING THE DOG
WALKING AFTER EATING
CHANGING EATING HABITS TO ASSIST COLONIC CANCER SURGICAL INTERVENTIONS
EXERCISE: SWIMMING, BEGINNING FACIAL MUSCLE CONTROL MOVEMENTS
LEARNING TO RELAX AND PRACTICE BREATHING
INCREASE NAPS TO MAINTAIN GOOD SLEEP

RHYTHMIC BREATHING
CENTAURING THROUGH ART AND MEDITATION
PRACTISING THE "WALKING TALK"
THIRD NATURE

CANCER, PARKINSONS DEMENTIA, SURGICAL INTERVENTIONS ACCIDENTS

SECOND NATURE

CHANGING ENVIRONMENT
NO STAIRS, LOOSE RUGS, GRAB-BARS IN BATHROOMS, NIGHT LIGHTS
DOWN-SIZING

(48)

Thinking about the Meaning of Muscles

Begin by getting an evaluation of your physical history; you can do this yourself by asking your caregivers, doctors or anyone else involved at this level with you. Then it is a good idea to find a mentor to help you. If you are healthy, or you have had any past injuries or blood pressure issues properly assessed then Activity is your Oyster!

Given that our muscles are the levers of our bones, it follows that they are one of the fundamental sources of our movements. Without them the skeleton literally falls down; we cannot begin any movements without them, even a smile! The facial muscles get quite the workout every day; I know, as I see the tracks they make in my mirror! It's the bigger muscles of our core physiology that are not often looked at in the bathroom mirror that get left behind literally, when we sit down. By the time we get to mid adolescence we have begun adult muscle development which continues until around our mid-twenties. Once it has finished developing it is perfectly ready for the workload it was designed for, and if nothing happens, this amazing structural array of inter-connective tissue created for our structural integrity begins to disintegrate, little by little. This process is known as atrophy, but believe me it's no prize! The

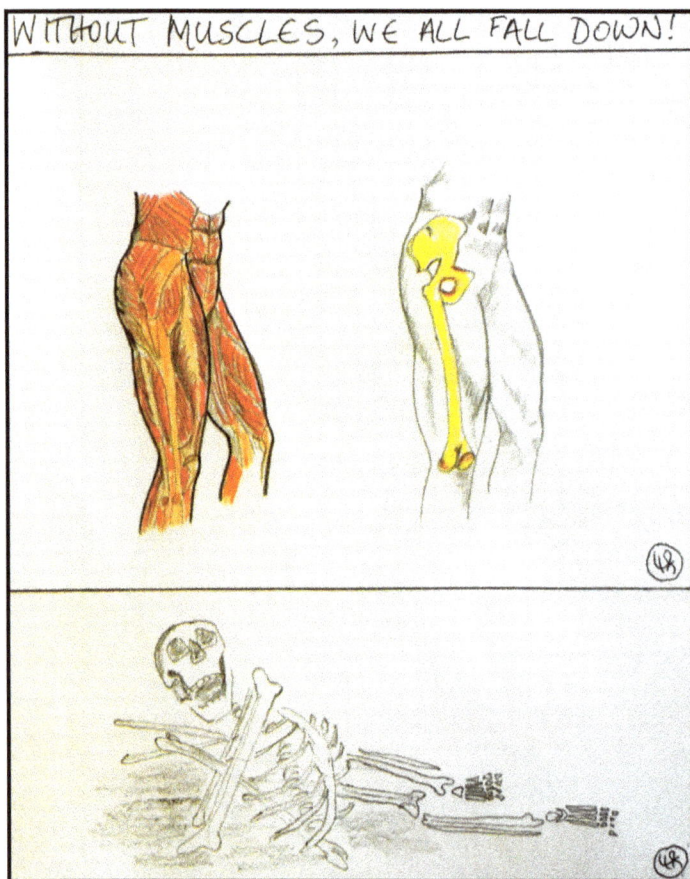

WITHOUT MUSCLES, WE ALL FALL DOWN!

muscle tone of youth sails south and the accompanying layers of skin sag without its underlying support system of muscle.

However, the magic of muscles is that we can call them back! We can rehabilitate them and give them a workload again and they will respond as they have a memory stored within their very cells; the key is activation! Strength training gives muscles back their primary functions. Muscles lift you up when you are going down, and they take you down in order to lift you up! We are not in the realm of superman, superwoman or competitive sports by the way. Muscles are one of the physical manifestations of Centauring yourself; in other words they keep you on your Horse! You cannot stand up without them, or breath, or even hold your head up. As an infant you spent half of your

AN EXAMPLE OF A "MASTER KEY" TO YOUR CENTAUR

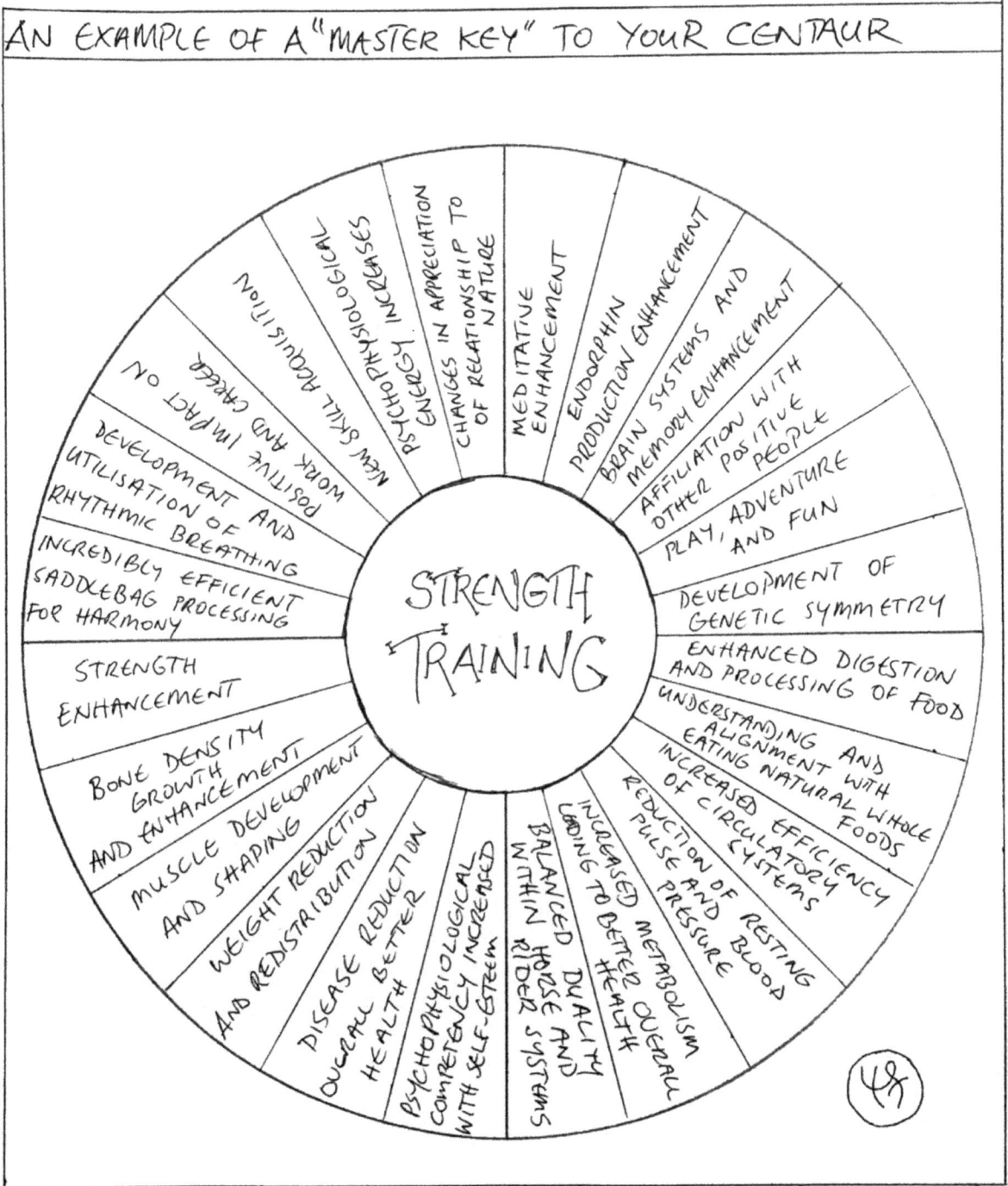

STRENGTH TRAINING

- MEDITATIVE ENHANCEMENT
- ENDORPHIN PRODUCTION ENHANCEMENT
- BRAIN SYSTEMS AND MEMORY ENHANCEMENT
- AFFILIATION WITH OTHER POSITIVE PEOPLE
- PLAY, ADVENTURE AND FUN
- DEVELOPMENT OF GENETIC SYMMETRY
- ENHANCED DIGESTION AND PROCESSING OF FOOD
- UNDERSTANDING AND ALIGNMENT WITH EATING NATURAL WHOLE FOODS
- INCREASED EFFICIENCY OF CIRCULATORY SYSTEMS
- REDUCTION OF RESTING PULSE AND BLOOD PRESSURE
- INCREASED METABOLISM LEADING TO BETTER OVERALL HEALTH
- BALANCED DUALITY WITHIN HORSE AND RIDER SYSTEMS
- PSYCHOPHYSIOLOGICAL COMPETENCY INCREASED WITH SELF-ESTEEM
- DISEASE REDUCTION OVERALL BETTER HEALTH
- WEIGHT REDUCTION AND REDISTRIBUTION
- MUSCLE DEVELOPMENT AND SHAPING
- BONE DENSITY GROWTH AND ENHANCEMENT
- STRENGTH ENHANCEMENT
- INCREDIBLY EFFICIENT SADDLEBAG PROCESSING FOR HARMONY
- DEVELOPMENT AND UTILISATION OF RHYTHMIC BREATHING
- NO IMPACT ON WORK AND CAREER
- NEW SKILL ACQUISITION
- PSYCHOPHYSIOLOGICAL ENERGY INCREASES
- CHANGES IN APPRECIATION OF RELATIONSHIP TO NATURE

113

life practicing using your brand new muscles! You were strength training with body weights before you even knew you were.

Classical shapes emanate from having muscles. The saddlebags, with which we can only make our way through this life with, are lighter if we have muscles to move us through the bad times, the sad times and into better times.

Healthy longevity relies upon movement and movement relies upon our muscle strength.

We all have some postural weakness that our muscles can either hinder or help with, and these are in the province of the stable master's help we suggested you find above.

Some examples could be:

Weak back muscles can mean a weak chest with a lessened capacity for full breathing, along with neck and head pains.

Weak leg muscles can mean lower back, hip, knee, and ankle troubles.

Weak stomach muscles will mean lower back issues.

There are a myriad of interconnected mechanic issues stemming from every muscle you own which can be partially responsible for how you are experiencing your Horse now but which, with proper interpretation can lead you to incredible changes with your Horse.

Don't compare yourself with others if it undermines your confidence, accept your own uniqueness and abilities as different to everyone else. In the playground at school most children did not wander around not playing because someone else looked better than they did!

The negative energy of comparison pops the delight of the movement moment.

Make a graded movement plan using stepping stones.

Walking on a flat surface for 30 minutes.

Walking with stairs and hills.

The "Peri-Odyssey" of Seasonality; Seasons of Energy

The most exciting thing about movement is that it has endless opportunities for variety. The chance for change is written into the whole way this planet operates on its great elliptical loop around our Sun. We call it a year, and we call them the seasons and they are designed to give us different energies at different times.

Have you ever noticed that the whole organic world has seasons of energy? Every living thing has bursts of energy, for example, plants have flowers which are then followed by what seems to be a dormancy that allows for the gathering of a renewed energy.

Summer, with its warmth and length of sunlight, allows for a lot more activity over longer periods of time. Many sports are commenced in the summer and people are more often found in outdoor pursuits; it is a time of enormous productivity.

Autumn with the days get a little cooler, and a little shorter, calls for activity to slow down in the natural world. We start to notice the difference quite markedly, and this brings with it the chance to assess the weather, its effects on us and to make adjustments to when and how we exercise.

Winter brings with it days that are darker and much shorter; the cold begins to bite and it's far more difficult for us to get up in the cold and race to the gym or into a morning activity. We want to sleep in more, to cuddle up in the blankets and rest in our nest. Our eating patterns involve more comfort foods as a response to the climatic change. The longer the winter is, in different regions of our world, the more likely that SAD (seasonal affective disorder), makes its mark felt. It is not easy when we are living in the dark to see how the light of getting up to exercise and move lifts our day and helps us to process those saddlebags! As a part of the natural world, our own psychophysiological system is geared towards more rest, in order to cope with the cold and dark, just as is every other mammals; not forgetting those other animals which go so far as to hibernate in their winter!

Spring brings with it the lengthening of the daylight hours and warmer temperatures allows the wakeup call of renewed energies from our rising sap! Our exercise patterns can be changed again to include a greater variety of longer activities.

Understanding the seasonal energy rhythms and patterns and then adapting and developing cyclic methods of movement and exercise based on this natural order of movement, will help to positively modify your ability to keep and maintain an on-going regular exercise programme all year round with a minimised risk of you overdoing it!

For woman especially, understanding your own personal monthly menstrual cycle of ebb and flow in these sorts of energy terms, can really contribute to having a much greater self-care opportunity which would otherwise be overlooked in an ongoing exercise regime.

Recovery Rewards

Resting after exercise is often misunderstood as a tool of movement as it is an exercise within itself. The more intense the type of exercise you choose to do on a regular basis, the more important resting afterwards becomes for the recovery of your HR system and for the avoidance of injuries and over-training.

Exercising in different seasons brings with it a biorhythmic opportunity to synchronise with the natural order of life and any opportunities we can create for ourselves through understanding our Natures in the light of this synchronisation with Life is something never to be ignored!

Spring and Summer bring opportunities for more energetic activities over the longer periods of daylight, while Autumn and Winter bring with them the need for a change of intensity to support our immune system's ability to adjust to harsher seasonal changes.

As we understand this, and from it develop the most natural, enjoyable and regular exercises we can choose for ourselves, it follows that an intrinsic "knowing" will become a part of our process. Then, from this understanding comes the learning that movement exercises themselves need to change over time; not only in tune with the seasons, but also in sympathy with our need to maintain an interest in them and to expand our motivation to continue doing them.

Just because we discovered in Chapter 2, that we are in this configuration, our HR duality, in order to cope and succeed with the adversities we face in our lives; it does not mean that while we are processing our saddlebags, and detoxifying their sometimes difficult contents, that we can't enjoy ourselves!

In fact, if we don't have fun and play in the world, which we have also discovered is absolutely necessary for our Horse child self, we will not manage adversity at all!

So, rather than burn out, in intense repetitive short-term activity, it stands to reason that for any long term ability to undertake our chosen, regular exercises, we need to take a more moderate and holistic approach.

Planning regular changes, in synchronicity with the seasons in the intensity and length of exercise programmes making sure to build in rest and relaxation, gives your HR system, your psychophysiology, the endurance it needs to go further for longer.

Injury undermines body and mind, draining away motivation for movement, the more positive the mind body energy you can muster for the task, the more you can achieve, as you are probably aware of in any activity situation.

Understanding Repressed Stress Symptoms

The tense moments in which we wait for things to happen or not happen, can in themselves, mount up and threaten to defeat us and are best described as negative kinetic energy.

Channeling this energy out of our HR system using the rhythm of movement, gives us an opportunity to create a positive from a negative; a bit like the theory of the universe beginning with a Big Bang, but perhaps a little quieter and less messy! This is nothing less than the psychophysiologic of your HR system working at its best for you. The cost of making your way, even successfully, through this life is paid for via the accumulation of such negative energies in our saddlebags. This will eventually drag us down under its weight and toxicity if we simply try and live with it. The conscious work which we can do to harness our HR system, our duality itself lessens both the effects of any toxicity and also the baggage weight too. You can harness the tension, the anger and any of the other energies and put them to work into activities that add to your life through the higher defence mechanism of sublimation. This process alone can positively influence not only your fitness levels but also your relationships, and it can add to the variety of movement opportunities you might have as well as outdoor travels. The ability to channel and master negative energy is a gift that keeps on giving.

Playgrounds of Adulthood

The world is full of chances for adult play, it's a jungle gym out there! We can take these chances and make a choice to initiate a takeaway of our own, in the form of the toxic waste of the day, and evaporate it into the positive energy sphere! That's not a bad reward that we get repaid by our Centaured being. After a bad day at work, you don't have to go home and "kick the cat" or have a fight with your partner; start obsessing about buying something new to feel better with; minimise reality, or drink to numb yourself, or consume horrendous junk foods, and in general blame anyone or anything else. This in fact is a wonderful chance to add so many positives, to rethink ideas, issues and problems to come up with better solutions and outcomes, and your loved ones will love you for it. To start the day again Centaured in the positive allows us the space to have capacity for concern for others, because we have taken the opportunity to care about our internal family first!

You can give your presence when you get present, or as G.I Gurdjieff once said: "Life is real, only then, when "I am".

Working forty five hours a week and then taking work home for the evenings and the weekend, a young professional couple tried to take a much needed break from work about every four months. They planned to have a week off, to help with work load stress levels and it meant they could have time alone together. What they found was, that as soon as their mini-break began, at least within a day or two, both of them had flu like symptoms and they felt quite sick. Their nerves felt frayed and they were depressed and irritable for almost all of their week off. They bickered and sulked and as soon as they returned to work they both felt a lot better. Of course, long gone was the much sort after rest, relaxation and romantic couple time that they had craved. A toxic buildup of inactivity, a takeaway diet and a difficult and stressful workload was kept stored psychophysiologically in their saddlebags. This bomb was released into their bloodstreams as soon as they left the defenses of their castle: the denial, minimisation, over eating, obsessional over working and their addictive reliance on the marvelousness of a large coffee stimulant in their morning and the delightful alcohol as a sugar relaxant in the evenings. Their combined psychophysiological systems Let Go of the negative energy poisons at each other; this noxious gas which was released into the atmosphere of their relationship spun it around and around in a spiral only down.

The Magnetic Negative

Have you ever had one of those days when everything seems to go wrong? Sometimes we walk into a maul (mall), and if feels like every other person is making a beeline with their weaponry, the enormous metal battering rams affectionately known as shopping trolleys, which we are given upon entry, straight into you? Call me paranoid, but it happens! In fact, it happens so much, that in my discussions with people, I have decided to give "it" a name. I call it the "magnetic negative", the definition of which is simple: it happens when you feel that negative energy seems to be attracted to you in large amounts in one way or another and you just can't catch a break. This in turn can take a reasonable day and a positive mood and turn it into a series of unfortunately irritable experiences.

When you discover that this is happening, it comes down to picking your battles; is it fight or flight, in which order, and with what intensity?

The spiral of the magnetic negative can produce hyper vigilance in us about the next difficulty we might encounter: the natural world is full of thorn bushes, bee stings, rocks to stub toes on, grass to be allergic to, cold places, hot places, sharks, spiders, snakes (we do live in Australia!), not to mention the psychological difficulties one has: bad drivers, difficult bosses, not enough rest, headaches, internet rip offs, it's all there and our Horse and Rider are now about as far away from their possible experiences of Third Nature as they could ever get!

Of course it is always dependent on the 1 – 10 scale of issue we have already visited and the ensuing choice of which reaction to what it's about and why. We remember the practice of using the higher defenses such as humour, friendship, asking for help, self-care preservation, meditative calming, along with the physical releases of the walking and talking techniques and these will change the energy around these situations.

The Yin and Yang of Pain, or using One kind of Pain to Resolve the Original Pain

Anyone who has had good remedial massage will know that it can be quite painful to unknot muscle and tissue in order to unlock blocked negative energies. We still, given all of the above which we have familiarised ourselves with in this chapter, sometimes need to undergo a naturally painful process to resolve the unnatural pain from which we are suffering.

As I have often said throughout this book, we are always geared towards avoiding the feeling of pain whether it is emotional or physical. That is, unless the payoff is an immensely gratifying one such as giving birth. Taking up a regular exercise activity does require a certain amount of consistent effort to develop a threshold that will facilitate growth and mastery. Starting with a commitment to one day at a time and breaking down the effort into smaller sets of movements builds a foundation to progress upon. No one starts a sport playing top level AFL or American Football or is an instant Olympian, just as learning a trade or the piano takes time, your body takes time to build as well, both internally, as in its lung capacity, muscle strength, and endurance as well as externally in its muscle size and silhouette.

Final Reflections

As in all things, mirrors too can be figurative; the mirror of our mind or literally, the mirror on the wall. Mirrors have been used in fairy stories and myths as archetypes reflecting all manner of human troubles. The Greek myth of Narcissus had a young and handsome man who fell in love with his own reflection in a pool of water, which eventually led him to become trapped beside the pool for so long that he turned into a the flower which now bears his name and is to be forever found growing in wet places. This is a good example of a cautionary tale about reflections; as is the story of Snow White, wherein the mirror is asked "mirror mirror on the wall, who is the fairest of them all?" Whether we are caught up adoring the perceived external beauty of ourselves or competing with others for the "most beautiful" title, this is Second and First Nature only. The fundamentally true mirror that Third Nature gives us is a reflection of the immutable laws of unceasing change in the natural world. Both First and Second Natures will change and be changed by these natural laws even though our survival instincts crave and clamour for no change at all, maintenance of the status quo. We cry for a lost youth, but deep within us, our higher energies crave the wisdom for change. This yearning is the yearning of our Centaur.

SELF HEALTH MEASUREMENT CHART

Psychological – Rider axis (upward progression):

- SEEK OUT A MENTOR FOR GUIDANCE
- OBTAIN AN OVERVIEW OF YOUR PHYSICAL AND MENTAL HEALTH
- TAKE PHOTOS. MAKE AN EXERCISE PLAN. FEEL YOUR SENSE OF PURPOSE
- FIND A TRAINING PARTNER, COUPLE OR GROUP - KEEP A RECORD
- LEARN TO CHANGE EXERCISE PROGRAMS INCREASING DIFFICULTY
- PERSONAL KNOWLEDGE INCREASES OF EXERCISE REGIMES THAT WORK
- DEVELOP REWARD SYSTEM FOR SELF-ESTEEM
- ATRUISTIC ABILITY TO PASS ON KNOWLEDGE
- CENTAURED
- GLOWING IN HEALTH, JOY, VITALITY AND EXCITEMENT

Physiological – Horse axis (upward progression):

- CHANGE CHOSEN - MAKE AN ACTION PLAN -
- START WALKING
- START CALORIES AS FUEL
- MODIFY YOUR FOOD SOURCE CALORIES, RUNNING, STRETCHING, SWIMMING
- CHANGE EXERCISES WORKING FOR YOU, NOT AGAINST YOU!
- BEGIN TO ADD IN OTHER PHYSICAL ENERGY
- NOTICE THE CHANGE IN YOUR PHYSICAL MOTIVATION ALONG - FOOD IS WORKING FOR YOU, NOT AGAINST YOU!
- START TO LOOK FORWARD TO PARTNER-SHIP AND MOTIVATION WITH SUPPORT
- FITNESS AND FRIENDSHIP DEVELOP THROUGH SHARED INTERESTS. COUPLE RELATIONSHIPS STRENGTHENED
- GAIN STRENGTH AND AEROBIC ENDURANCE
- ABILITY TO EXERCISE WITHOUT PARTNER, GROUP OR MANNER
- DEVELOPMENT OF INTRINSIC MOTIVATION
- CHANGES IN PHYSICAL DEVELOPMENT AND MENTAL ARE NOTICED BY OTHERS GIVING POSITIVE FEEDBACK
- HEALTH IMPROVEMENT NOTICED
- SYMMETRY BEGINNING TO BE GAINED
- GAINS REALLY BEGIN TO BE NOTICED
- ABILITY TO EXPLORE MANY DIFFERENT MOVEMENT FORMS AND EXERCISES
- VERY POSITIVE SELF-ESTEEM
- PSYCHOPHYSIOLOGY IS AT IT'S PEEK AND THE ABILITY TO EXPRESS OUR CENTAUR IS AT ONE OF IT'S PEAKS

Axes:
O PSYCHOLOGICAL - RIDER -
PHYSIOLOGICAL - HORSE -

FRANK'S STORY

'Leading horses to water and drinking deeply,
or always learning something new?'

Thirty years of strength training including a few competitions, working in gyms and training around other symmetrical sorts of sports people. Gave me a thirst for knowledge about how to make the benefits of investing in health work long term, in other words can I hang on to this physicality as I age? *(See photo of me at 24 yrs... yes, that is 1980's hair!)*

Thirty two years later I googled Frank Zane, a master trainer in San Deigo U.S,A. who at 73 yrs of age had been strength training for 60 years. He had won many competitions, written many books on the subject of muscle and fitness and was running courses in Body building, longevity wholistic health. His whole adult life dedicated to maintaining and teaching muscle symmetry fitness in a harmonious balance whatever age one may be.

Being part of a couple I wanted health to be our health, so when I met my husband Michael our circles became a ring of steel forged together working out with weights, taking journeys together in gyms for 20 years. We discussed having a mentor and looking for inspirational motivation for moving forward in functional health and well being, making the most of what we had gained from our exercises. We were going to San Diego California for good vibrations!

Frank after meeting us says he wants to take our pictures and photoshop them creating some interesting effects! Next day; wow! What an epiphany, after 30 years of thinking we were on to it, Frank really surprised us. His philosophy of visual-isation based on the objectivity of the photos really opened our eyes to what we could achieve.

We had been focused on our wholistic health for 30 years using body-building as a central strut and we thought we had been doing pretty well, knowing we didn't

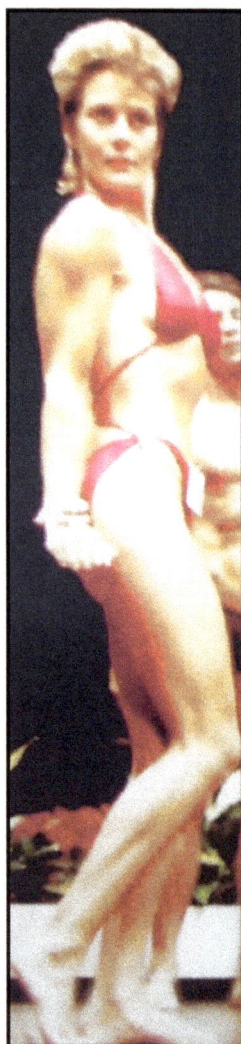

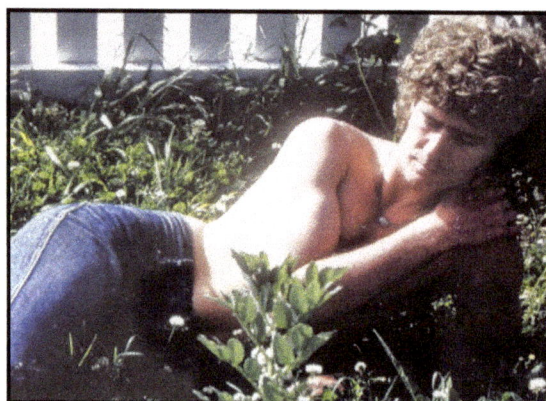

Michael straight out of the Garden of Eden. 19 yrs old contemplating life after representative rugby.

know it all but Frank's master class has helped us into renewed gains, health and success.

Traveling over S.E.Asia for our work for the past 10 years has forced us to scrutinise food very closely, especially protein. As we have aged, both of us have experienced what seemed to be reactions to whey products, we were looking smooth or even puffy so we changed to plant protein but were not really feeling it was right either. Meeting Frank and listening to his vast experience switched us on Day 1 to get into his Egg White Perfection and it has been simply the best protein we have ever used in our lives. After 2 months using it the difference is obvious and these pictures are taken pre-workout and without any photo shopping.

Frank's expertise and critique has given us a whole new focus and vision for our workouts: radically cutting back on our carbs and fats and changing our protein to egg white perfection.

(See photos)

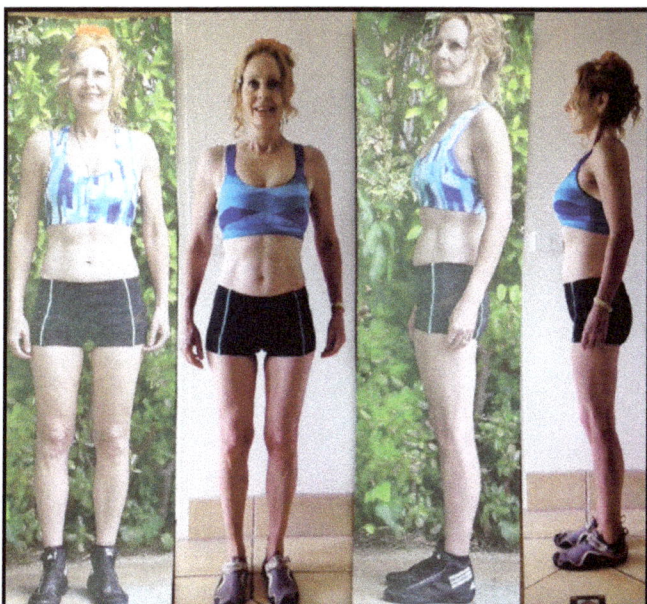

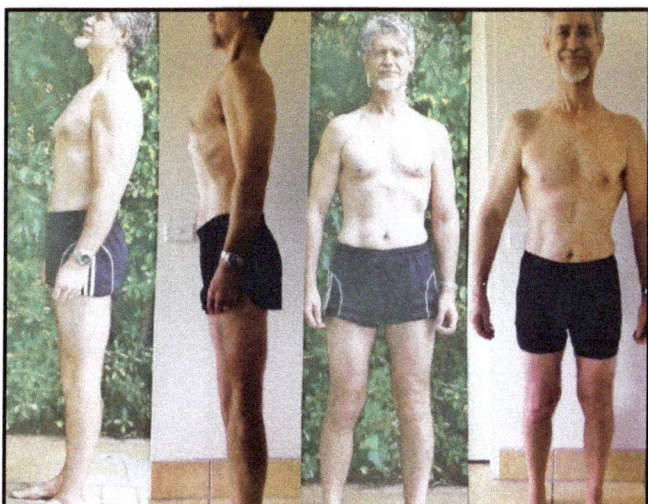

We changed our workouts to follow his silhouette philosophy developing our deltoids and calves while shrinking the waistline and maintaining as much muscle overall as possible.

Our workout principles however are best described by Frank in his book "Let's Grow" 2014.

We are currently doing one of the four 3 way splits he describes called "Let's Grow Routine" consisting of :

Day 1: back, rear and side delts, triceps and abs

Day 2: legs and abs

Day 3: chest, front delts, biceps, forearms and of course abs

This routine has really begun to work on the stubborn areas which have not responded as well to past routines.

My waistline has diminished and my pecs, delts and lats have all grown while my weight has remained the same. Michael's lower abs, waistline and overall body fat have all diminished while retaining and growing calve and upper body muscle.

We have only seen these changes

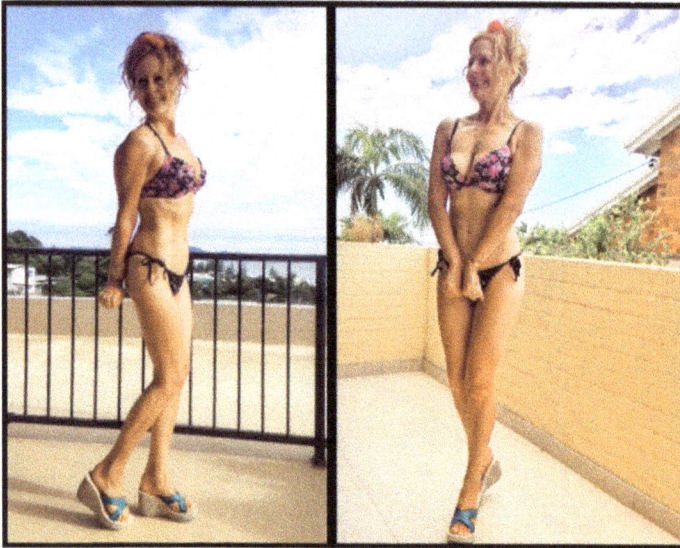

Sara at 55 with absolutely no Photoshop.

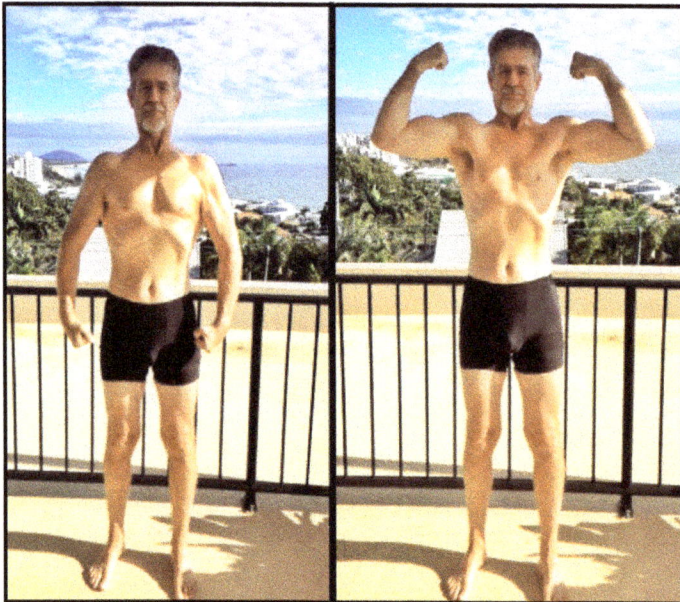

Michael at 58 with absolutely no Photoshop.

as clearly because we followed Frank's direction and have been taking photos to compare progress. In addition we have been using visualisation and meditation techniques prior to our workouts.

One of the other remarkably simply yet effective changes within our workouts has been stretching between every set. This has added the dual benefit of keeping the muscles warm between sets and giving them the best recovery

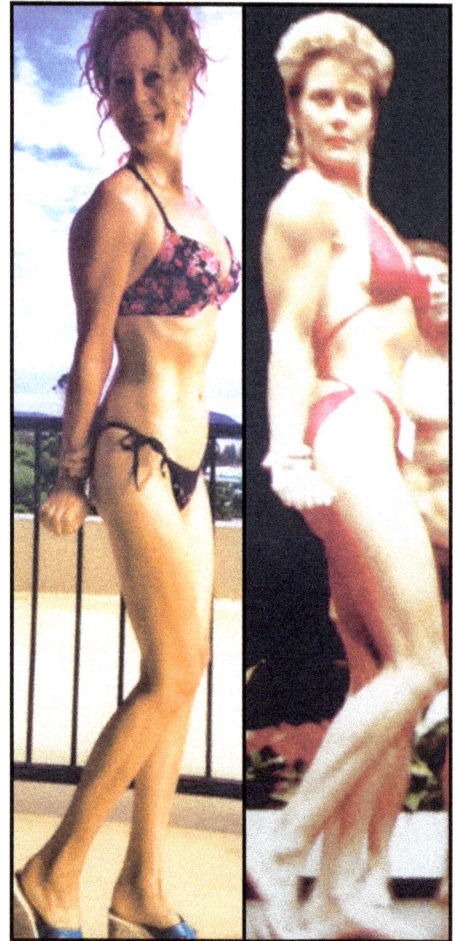

Posing: The Final Frontier

possible through stretching so they can come back at their best for the next and subsequent sets. While we were stretching somewhat before in our workouts we were never really, it turns out, giving ourselves the best opportunities in the workout we could.

We have now, as of this week, taken up yoga as a

part of our aerobic routine.

Frank taught us that it's not enough just to have muscles, you have to be able to use good posture for your body silhouette to its best advantage as you see here and in the posture photos.

This mentoring experience gave us an incredible energy boost in our mid and later 50's; the critique and support of our bodybuilding journey lives with us every day and has revolutionised our goals and vision for the coming years. We can hang on to our physicality longer, take our health further than I ever thought possible in 1984!

The positive psychological impact of seeing the gains initially portrayed in the first photos and then again in the photos we took so soon after switching proteins really blew us away. When we used a better protein source, added up the calories and put in more supplements, meanwhile fine tuning our workouts then took a final set of photos, the progress is obvious and spurs us on to continue and increase our focus.

Seeing is believing, a truly centuring outcome!

This mentoring opportunity has been worth every cent we spent getting from one side of the planet to the other and meeting Frank has been one of the highlights of our lives!

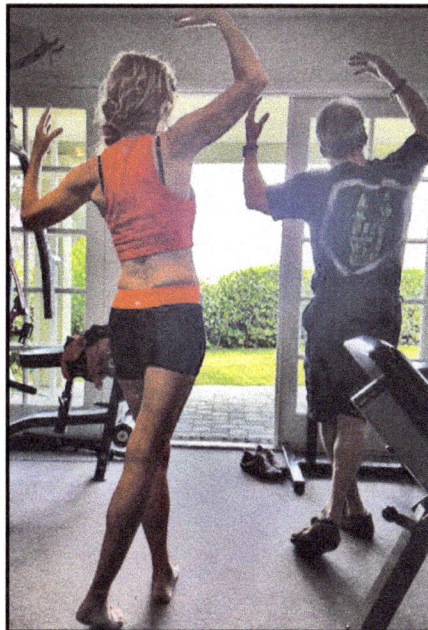

Gita Bellin: 'The impossible is possible when people align with you; when you do things with people, not against them, the amazing resources of the higher self are mobilised.'

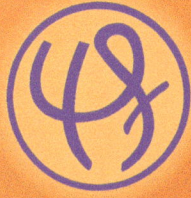

CHAPTER 6

THIRD NATURE

'We were energy before we mattered.'

Sara Beaumont-Connop

'An atemporal being   (Centaur)
Manifesting an organic body   (Horse)
Experiencing metaphysical states.'   (Rider)

We have traveled together through this book, investigating what is actually a part of our self-knowledge, but which nevertheless, quite a few of us have forgotten. In Chapter 4 Horse and Rider learn to eat together again instead of alone, split from each other's uniquely symbiotic energies. They learn to eat for three, feeding their Centaur. In Chapter 5 Horse and Rider are introduced to each other's energies through the harmonious movement and enjoyment of that movement again. Rider thrills to the feel of the Horse's strengths and abilities and Horse loves being given what it so aches for and needs and is guided by the Rider. The infinity number is represented as the pathway changing the negative kinetic energies which are an inevitable byproduct of passing through this life and its adversities, into the sometimes hard worked for, but passionately experienced positive energies. It is through this process that we can find ourselves expressing and experiencing our Centaur.

Every day is a new day; we can't have yesterday back and tomorrow is not present yet. We are left in this moment, to choose what we will do with this day, the day we have to live our lives in. You know that you can have a focused work plan, if this is a work day as they don't usually pay you just for showing up. So how can you, on this day, take the best holistic care of yourself, with all of the opportunities you do have, how does this Centauring work?

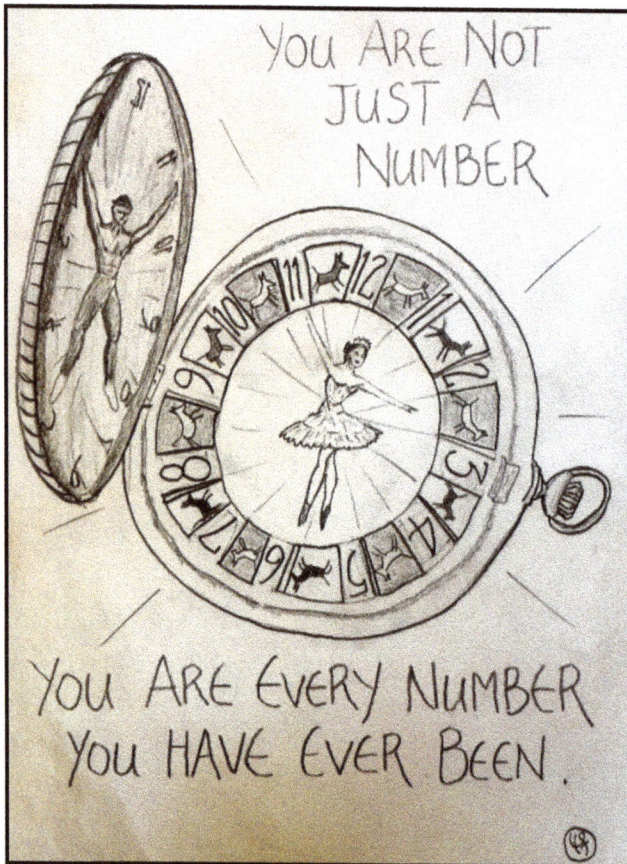

You ARE NOT JUST A NUMBER

You ARE EVERY NUMBER YOU HAVE EVER BEEN.

The goal is always to take what you do have and work with it to capture The Conscious Moment. Consciousness in the moment is the focus of your two energies in relation to an idea, a state of being, a problem you want to resolve, anything in short which you wish to work on. The first energy is that of hindsight and the second, that of insight. When these two sights are coupled they can produce a third energy, that of an external combined with an internal force we call foresight. This looks like the infinity symbol, the figure 8 we have met before when looking at changing negative kinetic energies into the positive processing energy we need in our HR configuration.

Centauring is the balance of First and Second nature, which enables our higher mind the space and ability to create something greater than what is already past or present. It is the timeless opportunity to gain inspiration about one's being and life. Where you come from, where you are, and where you want to go. It is not a religion nor is it magical thinking. It is using the creative higher energy of love. Energy is always on a spectrum of negative to positive and we are concerned with the most positive creative energy that there is in the human experience; it's the same kind of brilliant electrical spark that brought your life into this organic realm.

This emanated from the unconditional love or the love that was "good enough", from your caregivers for the new life they created; and as we saw back in Chapter 1, we know you would have died through a failure to thrive without it. So, all of the imagined, and then realised love actions, that your caregivers gave you, teaching you to walk and talk, to master your universe; came from this ultimately altruistic energy that lifted you up from your cradle and into the circle of arms that held you in positive regard. This love, mixed with your own unbelievable determination to stand and move into your world enabled you to take your place Centaured within yourself. This balancing of your psychophysiological energies worked to create the love bond attachment between your caregiver and you and it has a quality, an energy signature. That love then became the motivational force for you to achieve all the milestones of growth towards adulthood.

All of the balancing of your mind and body's energies that you practiced growing up, now dwells within you. These, in themselves have given rise to your own ability to care for, create and manifest your individual self-determination. It is not only the wish and creation of children that comes from this dimension of higher mind; we can focus on any creative endeavour using this positive well-spring, when harmony reigns between the psychophysiological self.

Many famous people such as, Nelson Mandala, Charles Dickens, Michelangelo and Walt Disney have used this higher mind consciousness to design and create great things for the benefit of humanity while tapping into the Centaured self in the fully conscious moment.

Being peacefully present in our HR duality means that energy can flow to our higher thought processes enabling the creative engagement of possibilities when we are dealing with adversity. Using the three sights, we can achieve change there, conceiving ideas that we may not have been able to think of in times of tension.

Imagine this: you living are in a small town in the desert and there is a terrible drought. No one has enough water, nothing will grow as there is no irrigation, everyone is thirsty, hungry and angry. You look at your neighbours with avarice in your eyes, as you feel depleted and deprived. When your neighbour's child dies, you have no tears for them as you are shriveled and hard from suffering and so you do nothing. When your own child dies, your neighbour also does nothing. No one in the town survives, because no one did anything to change the situation. Over the sand dune there is another you who lives in the same conditions, however this you takes the walking talk energy and tries to imagine solutions to the town's problems. This you, then enlists their neighbours help and so on, until the whole town engages to discuss possible solutions. The idea of using divination to locate and dig a well comes into your mind and the others agree to help. The positive energy of the motivated group is harnessed into the activity. The gushing well fast becomes the Centaur of the town square and the town is saved.

The Three Wishes Exercise

In the therapeutic setting children are given the opportunity to have three imaginary wishes to think about what could be. Naturally this engenders wishes for more wishes or millions of dollars, but not as often as you would think! Eighty percent of the wishes that I have witnessed being wished for, over a twenty year period have most often been for changes in relationships and situations. Often children have great insight into their problems, but little chances to effect change.

That is what the therapy was for; to help the child reconnect with their family in an insightful and caring way. The use of hindsight and understanding into what had gone wrong in the relationships, or the situation causing any problems to be enacted by the child, and projected onto themselves, the family or the school environments was the cornerstone of any successful therapeutic corroboration. We could then formulate active interventions with parents, caregivers and the child to bring about holistic changes. If you were able to put aside the greed wishes of the material world and be honest about what you truly wish for, what would those 3 wishes be? Try to prioritise them in order from most important to least; you may surprise yourself.

How do we elicit a goal from our imagination and then create it in our reality? If we were to ask this of any Olympian or famous person they would most likely talk about these things:

Motivations and Rewards

There are three types of motivation for any behavior;

	Intrinsic Motivations	
FIRST NATURE	SECOND NATURE	THIRD NATURE
MONEY	FOOD	BELIEF AND FAITH
SELF RESPONSIBILITY	RELATIONSHIPS	ACTUALISATION
SELF COMMITMENT	SELF ESTEEM	CREATIVITY
FUN	PLAY	PASSION
SELF SACRIFICE	GAINS	VISUALISATION
ALTRUISM	INTIMACY	LOVE

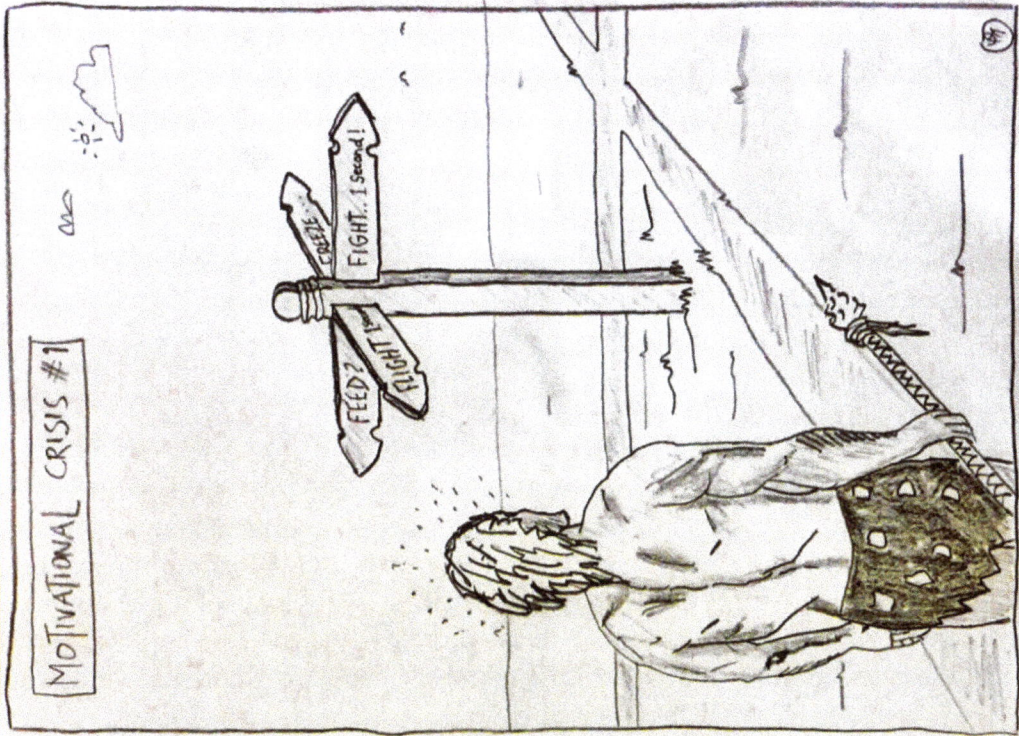

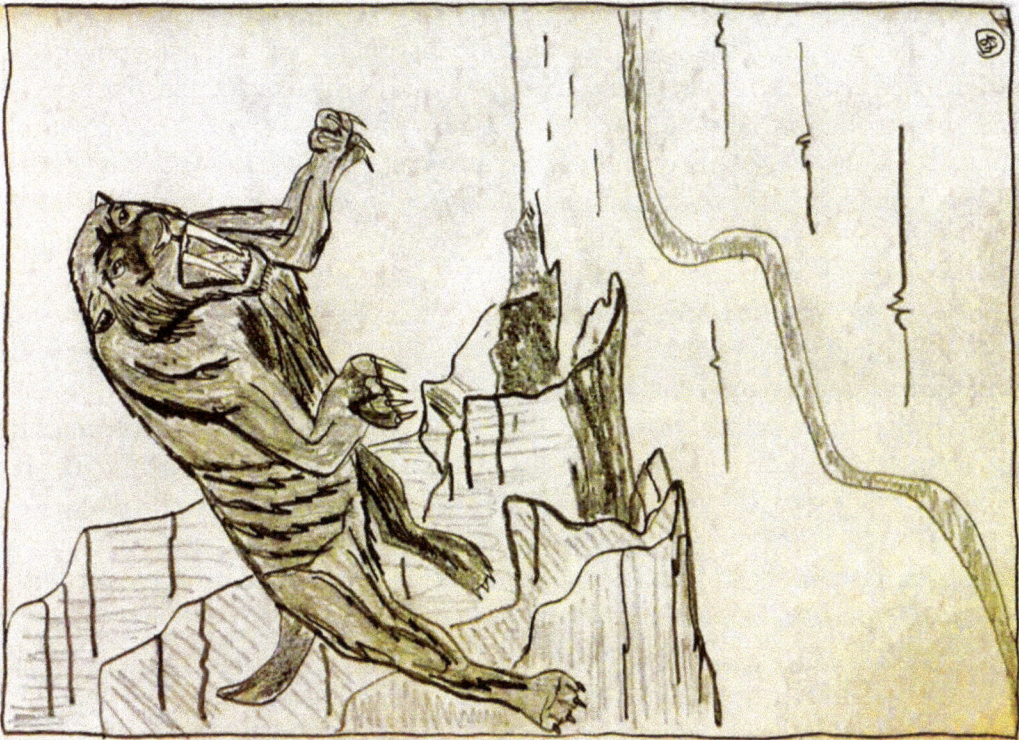

Motivators are an indispensable part of the journey to our Centaur, and in the wider context of this journey, we are moving to balance the first two varieties in order to achieve the third, and through this, Centaur ourselves. We may use the external motivators such as rewarding ourselves after movement with a planned enjoyable snack or new gym shoes, in order to satisfy our First and Second Natures, because we are what we are! However our goal is to move from these external motivators and engage our internal motivators. If, for example, you can't train with a partner or group you can still feel positive enough not to give up your movement, because you feel inspired to do it for the psychophysiological pay off; the sheer joy of knowing, through experiencing your essential oneness with Nature.

Being Centaured does not mean being perfect!

Change precludes perfection

Perfection is the ability to change

Nothing living stands still unchanging

Life is changing moments in movements

It is much more a process of "how you take the changes" and what you do with them.

There was once a king in a far off land, whose wife died giving birth to their only child, a daughter. The baby was perfect in every way, except for a large strawberry birthmark covering the right side of her face but the king loved his daughter. As she grew up the princess was everything kind and good, however the king made her wear a veil coronet, for he knew, that others would only see her birthmark and judge her for its curse on her beauty. Then the day came when the king knew the princess needed to marry for the good of the kingdom, and so he sent out riders to spread the word amongst all the royal princes. Many came, as the king was very rich and the kingdom powerful. The first suitor arrived and came to see the princess; the princess lifted the veil from her face and the prince's face registered horror upon seeing the birthmark and he turned away and left. So it came to pass that each prince turned away and left after seeing the princess's marked face. Finally, after the last prince left, the princess took off her coronet veil, her jewels and her rich clothing. She dressed as a village maiden, called for her horse and out of the palace gates she rode, her birthmark blazing through the streets. She traveled over the whole kingdom, having many adventures and learning about her people. One day she came to a forest full of mystery and tall tales, and there in the middle of this forest, leaning against a tree, was a prince with his head bowed down, writing about his many journeys. At the sound of her approaching horse he looked up to see the princess slowly smiling at him and the prince smiled back, for the prince had the exact birth mark on the left side of his face as the princess had upon her right, they were a match. No, they did not return to the princess's father's kingdom, but travelled to distant shores and there on the highest cliff overlooking the vast universe of an ocean, the prince and princess built a new kingdom of their own, where difference really did make a difference in the lives of all those who inhabited it.

Remember the Language of your Body! Photos of the Mind, taken by the Body

The external, mirrors the internal, in a myriad of ways. For many years I worked with abused teenage girls and every day I put on my best suit or dress. I managed my hair into a style and put my earrings and makeup on. This type of dressing was not the norm for the district, but based on my experience of psychiatric patients and teenage young women's body language, I believed in representing hope, energy and care in my own body language, making it an active part of the treatment, other than just words. There were always comments about this presentation, people do see it and it does define what you are saying about yourself to others.

Getting a new haircut/style can be the most uplifting experience or the most humiliating.

Malnutrition of Third Nature

As we discussed in our very first chapters, a baby can be fed, warm and clean, however they can still fail to thrive and die. This death is a consequence of the inability of the caregiver to see beyond the psychophysiological into the force of nature that is the love attachment. The nourishment of this part of ourselves is the primary goal of this book. If we fail to see our need for this kind of sustenance, then a part of ourselves is unable to move as it is starved by the other two; drowned out by our bodies many cries for foods or our minds many cries for stimulants. The external world of human contrivances impinges upon this struggle with its environmental demands and expectations, projecting upon us in every way imaginable, looking to take our conscious attention and focus it on something serving its own purpose. The chance for nourishing that part of our self which thrives in the harmony of our balancing, and develops in the infinite conscious moment of Centauring is often far removed from our noisy human world. Try creating a constant noise over 85 decibels in a new born baby's nursery. Why is it that we need so much exterior noise to fill our interior self that already has its own natural noises? So far I have not been to a very loud yoga class, but I have had to put on noise cancelling head phones in a gym, just to hear myself think! Concentration and focus go hand in hand with movement. How loud does the engineered environment need to be before we are battered into feeling nothing, hearing nothing, and thinking nothing, senselessly lost in the sounds of others? This state of being is not a consciousness in the moment and does not lead to any centre, rather, it can only dull any awareness we might develop of our potential linkages to Third Nature.

Love with Boundaries or Self-care: The ability to delay gratification in the service of greater self actualisation.

There are two ways to create great difficulties in a child's life, the first is to give them nothing, to provide an environment of extreme deprivation. The second is to give the child whatever they want all of the time. This child with their every whim catered to, begins to feel entitled to whatever they want at any time and a needy, greedy cycle is set up. No matter how much this child is given, they will always want something bigger, better, and more of it. The fantasy of this child for example, is that they should win at everything, at any game and all of the time. This vicious circle can only lead to the frustrating disillusionment with reality, and the people that shaped their expectations in this manner; because somewhere out there, there is an inescapable loss waiting to happen, a tantrum of a want that cannot be satisfied; and the unfortunate series of adversities, which will take them down. We owe it to our inner child to have boundaries on how much of the material world we can consume, literally and figuratively. There has never been a time, so overwhelmingly deluged with opportunities to consume so much so easily. There are so many examples of so people, who have so many collections, of so much stuff packed into their saddlebags that they cannot fit it into their homes or garages and now second hand thrift shops do a roaring trade as they continue to move to ever expanding premises. Do we really believe that "more" of this is truely the answer?

Developing a caring discipline as a goal is something that schools strive for, because they know, that it is only in this circle, the boundary of caregiving, that children can learn to focus and the develop the ability to internalise good habits.

Quote: It is from the individual the group grows and within the group the individual grows.

No reasonable education system is unstructured to the point that there is no developmental growth philosophy. They are looking to enhance the best in their students, through the principles of love with boundaries. That, in a sense, is what you will achieve using your higher defence mechanisms of awareness, commitment and self actualisation.

So circles have a symbolic meaning in the universal consciousness of cultures throughout the world, for example the circle as a ring given at a wedding ceremony, representing eternal love. Where is the chance to commit to ourselves? If we put that beautiful, positive energy circle around ourselves, we have the chance to begin in the physical and end in the metaphysical, the joy of being, consciousness in the moment. One of the first steps allowing us to activate our Third Nature is the choice of a place for thoughtful contemplation. We call it the "development of the capacity to be alone", contained and at peace with the external and internal world we are in.

A very famous child psychiatrist and paediatrician walked into the lecture hall which was filled to overflowing with that countries best child specialists waiting to hear him talk. He walked up to a chalk blackboard without saying anything to his audience and drew the diagram you see below this. He then turned to his audience and asked any one of them to venture the meaning of the peculiar looking pictogram he had drawn. Not one of them guessed out loud for fear of making an error in front of their peers, let alone the man standing in front! See what you can make of it, remembering it is symbolic and the lecture he was giving was about the difficulties children have leaving the safety of the caregiver and venturing into the world!

This is the very same process that we all used to first gain the ability of exploring the world as children. All of the interactions between caregiver and child, involving the child checking the caregiver's loving care and it's continuance over the time the child is exploring are there. The child leaves and returns to the caregiver and the pattern is repeated, it creates a circle around the caregiver while the caregiver's holding love creates a circle around the child. The

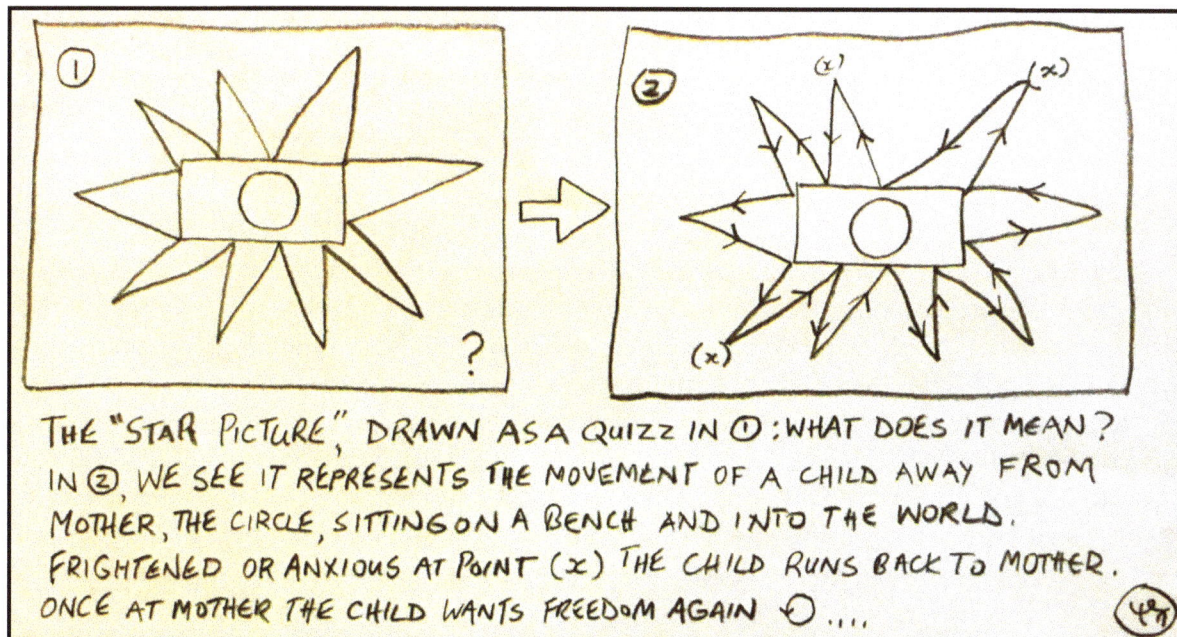

THE "STAR PICTURE", DRAWN AS A QUIZZ IN ① : WHAT DOES IT MEAN ? IN ②, WE SEE IT REPRESENTS THE MOVEMENT OF A CHILD AWAY FROM MOTHER, THE CIRCLE, SITTING ON A BENCH AND INTO THE WORLD. FRIGHTENED OR ANXIOUS AT POINT (x) THE CHILD RUNS BACK TO MOTHER. ONCE AT MOTHER THE CHILD WANTS FREEDOM AGAIN ⟲ ....

combination of these two evolving circles, each attached to each other, demonstrates the ability of the child to be in the world and alone for a while. This is the holding environment that the love of the caregiver provides to the exploring child. It holds them both psychologically and physically; it is the safety net that allows us the independence of spirit and courage to master our environment. We were facilitated and encouraged to do this. The more contained we felt the bigger the circles we could achieve, the bigger the circles were, the bigger the journeys we undertook; this is where the star, that you are, began!

We all learnt to combine our two natures, psychological and physical, Horse and Rider, to gain that positive energy between who we were and what we could do with who we were. Thoughts transformed into activities – Thinking – Talking - Doing.

You individuated because you could be alone, but internally you were never really alone. That lesson which you learnt doing the "star" process above, gained you the positive experiences that you collected in your mind and body as you were exploring your world. These experiences and their internalisations sustained you on your path, walking, running, jumping, angry, happy, sad; and then you went home for the love energy that was accepting and glad of your being.

Now all of this collected, remembered and stored energy is at your command. All of those loving moments are there together with the capacity to be alone and explore the external world and the internal world of your thoughts and feelings. The capacity for care and concern that has become a part of you, is also within you there and can be accessed by the needs of your higher defence mechanisms to enable your mastery over tasks and adversities you face in your world.

Accessing Third Nature

How do we tap into this third nature that emanates harmoniously from the duality of your mind and body, your Horse and Rider energies?

Conscious Action: developing Foresight from Hindsight and Insight equals Centauring.

Movement provides a physical energy, an input balancing the internal and external. Sitting, passive energy with the standing active energy $-----$ and $||||||=+$; a positive!

The bioelectrical energies transcending from the activated psychophysiologic systems engages and transforms us, providing the spontaneous ability to create and inspire. Dickens created his stories walking around London and Freud, Nietzsche and Schopenhauer theirs, walking around Vienna, Heidelberg and the Black Forest.

You will often garner information about your energy's alignment from comments you receive from other people, like: "you're looking great, up for it, healthy and well". The age you are has no "number" really; you can have a light and energy which flows from you no matter what "age" you are. This radiance of yours can be attained at any age and kept at any stage of your life cycle. It is seen naturally as a "glow" from pregnant women but it is also seen emanating from anyone who is Centauring.

The Conscious Moment: Stretching the Mind to Hear the Sounds of Self-Observation

Where do you go to when you are alone in your head? This can be one of the times when you are fully conscious in the moment of your higher self. Lending an inner ear to listen to these musings, gives rise to opportunities for creative thoughts, thoughts that differ from the everyday. Being in the natural world adds to the chance of being able to blend our first and second natures to find our Third.

The walking meditative thought, or, if with a friend, the walking meditative talk, aligns itself with your rhythmic breathing and is a beautiful background to then blend your hindsight over the issues concerning you. This exercise produces a timelessness within your conscious awareness that allows insight to arise in the presence of hindsight when analysing any issues. The frantic change of the external world falls away as this calm Centaur of self arises within you and your Third Nature provides foresight. This same state can be accessed just before falling asleep and one way you can assist it is to use the meditative breathing exercise outlined earlier in this book. It brings a great clarity and calmness of mind and when used as a guided visualisation it will allow the dissipation of intrusive thoughts that can disturb our minds inner sight and prevent us from accessing our Centaur of self.

It is this stretching of the mind that gives us an elasticity of spirit, gains us the resilience to endure adversity, and develops the flexibility to try new ideas and motions. Most great thinkers went to quiet places to reflect upon life, the world and their place in it. They practiced self observation using reflective thought, or in other words, hindsight coupled with the rising insight, to gain new information or different ways of seeing the same information based upon the behaviour and feelings only the individual can come upon.

You are the dream and you are the dreamer. You are the Horse and you are the Rider.

No one can really have the answers for you, because your reality is your own creation. It has been built by every choice, decision and experience that you have ever had. Your behaviours belong to you and your meaning for them is also ego syntonic to you. Others can interpret these for you however only you will truly know if they are right.

Your in sight is the gift that you have for sight into the life you lead and what you want from it!

Everyone has memories, billions of memories, but only you have your memories and your dreams for your life, so visualising in the conscious moment is your own unique tool for today enabling you to change tomorrow.

Stretching the Boundaries of Stretching

STRETCHING THE BOUNDARIES OF STRETCHING		
PHYSICAL	PSYCHOLOGICAL	CENTAURED
ORIENTATION IN THE ENVIRONMENT	RELAXATION OF THOUGHT	OPENED TO CREATIVITY
BREATHING IN RHYTHM	REFLECTION OF THOUGHTS	HARMONY
HINDSIGHT	INSIGHT	FORESIGHT
POSITIVE ENERGY FLOW	INTUITION	INSPIRATION

Couple Hood and the Hoods we Wear

Over the last five chapters we have covered babyhood, childhood, teenage hood, adulthood and parenthood in the pursuit of discovering Horse and Rider hood.

What we have been discussing throughout this journey is our attachment to others and ourselves, and out of this First Nature, the ability to be aware of ourself and the other. This awareness potentially grows into what we call the "capacity for concern" for others, and this in turn leads to the development of some of our highest defence mechanisms, those of altruism and the appreciation of the natural world, the environment we find ourselves coexisting in. The love that is talked about at wedding ceremonies is most often Third Nature in origin. It is the love that talks of an unconditional care and concern one for another. It is the love that makes promises of forsaking any self-serving actions for a greater good of the couple, whatever the circumstances. It is the love with which ushers in the beginning of a "new life", with all of the small steps that that life entails. It takes some time to learn to know one another's likes and dislikes, needs and wants. Just as a baby comes into the circle of the caregiver, so too do each partner in the couple circle take time to fill each other. Often they take turns at being the caregiver, developing the feelings of love, safety, sharing, and fun. Long term commitment grows and sets its roots and love through the use of our higher defence mechanisms. It needs energy and work in order to thrive, just as your being took the same path growing up. Our understandings of how and why we are in this particular configuration, which we have carved out for ourselves in the exploration of Horse and Rider, are completely applicable, naturally enough, to any relationship, whether it is a couple, group, community or society. So, for the couple it is the same as for the individual; we use our collective hindsight to develop our insight which gives rise to our Centauring foresight within the couple hood. When we begin a relationship, we begin it with a hope and a passion that the feelings and actions that we facilitate within the relationship will develop into a healthful partnership; a trusting and reliable way of living which will lead to creative opportunities, a home, perhaps travel, children, and of course shared interests. Long-term relationships always include health issues, let's face it, everyone gets the flu, becomes tired and occasionally has accidents. The phrase "in sickness and in health", is a phase that was in the past always uttered as a promise in wedding vows. It was there for a reason! One's health and sickness definitely comes into the "living together" scenario at some stage of the proceedings. Health impacts in serious ways upon the life of the relationship. No one is at their best in illness as it pulls us back to earlier times when we were more dependent upon others. This will strain the ability of any caregiver's capacity for concern if we are ill and unwell for repetitive or long periods of time.

In a Centaured relationship, the gift of sharing uplifting and playful activities which lead to healthful outcomes for both, give the relationship opportunities for growth, just as it does for the individual.

Centauring your Natures as a couple releases your Third Nature energies, which are inspirational, altruistic and committed to overcoming adversities together. This blending of both partners, each able to love and sustain the other, generates another appearance of the infinity symbol, the figure 8, and when that happens, you are truly Running with Rainbows!

These capacities for care and concern which are part of our higher being, are the love energies which we take in to account with the choice of our life partner. The ability to nurture one's self psychophysiologically allows for a much greater quality of love and care in other relationships, especially the person or people you choose to live your life with on a daily basis. Reflect for a moment on the idea of wanting the best health for the people you love, the best outcomes for their lives and for happiness, as a daily part of who they are. How does love achieve this? Remember right back in the beginning of this book, we talked about the moment by moment, day by day tasks, of interactional physical and psychological caregiving that the parent gave the infant? This interactional awareness of "the other" which caregiver and infant find in their relationship, has been called "intersubjectivity". There is a growing awareness of the other as the relationship deepens, and this deepening is where the delight in the other's being is found. The babies which survived through WW2 that Bowlby studied, survived because they were "found" by the other, in the form of a bond of care.

These same practices of love in the service of daily care can be extrapolated into the couple relationship. If each member of that relationship is actively aware of the other's needs, and makes an effort to facilitate both Horse and Rider activities promoting holistic health, then that relationship can be said to be well on the road to Centaured. Each of us requires caring love over our whole life-times, not just as a child or teen. The relationships we have within ourselves and others are the journey to our Centaurs; they are living energies, that within our conscious capacity for concern, grow deeper and more meaningful from our first breath to our last.

Third Nature gives us the ability to Live our Lives in the Infinite Moment at Full Speed.

> Quote: *There is Nothing…*
> *If YOU never*
> *Imagined,*
> *Dreamed,*
> *Believed,*
> *Said, or*
> *DID*
> *IT!*

Transcendental Humming - Taking the Path Less Travelled

The alignment of thought with movement, it is first a conscious decision to suspend impulsive actions in the service of making better choices and outcomes in situations that are difficult/stressful. It is a conscious focus upon making a space in your mind using the rhymic opportunity of breathing, walking, stretching and or exercising.

A realisation occurs that difficulty in thought is being experienced.

A pattern of behaviour is noted for example impulsive behaviours are occurring, inability to make concentrate on tasks and complete them.

A chance to get up and step away from the situation is given, a small time out.

Impulsive actions and panic thinking are delayed by making this decision.

Getting up and walking away breathing/stretching

Giving permission to hear yourself think.

Reflecting on the moment, (a quiet word in your inner ear), just do release of negative energy by rhymic action to calm the horse. To look in, for sight for options of being that create wellness in the use of the duality of psychophysiological in other words Use your horse to jump the hurdles together.

After 15-20 mins breathing/walking the higher mind has an opportunity to be heard, a positive attunement with self in the environment is attained. Creative ideas and opportunity.

In the modern world the Fight/Flight analogy cannot work in all situations

What about Crystal?

At the end there is always a beginning, even if we don't know what it will turn out to be. It is four years since Crystal phoned with her riderless horse in tow. What happened, did she get back up on her horse? Obviously Crystal had some changes to make. She stopped working at the call centre, her foot recovered and she moved into a boarding situation with family friends for a time. She then moved into another flat which she shared with her sister and another young woman. Crystal enrolled in a naturopathic course and started a part-time sales position in a health food shop which supported her gaining and using the naturopathy degree.

Crystal took the time to have her eyes checked by an optometrist and a photograph of her retina was taken. For the first time in her life, she really looked into her own eyes seeing the brilliantly detailed photographic images sparkling back at her. Twin universes, full of colour and beautifully dazzling energies. "Wow!" she thought, "That's me, they belong to me, I have whole physical world's that I have never even dreamed of, everything they do, is in the service of helping me, completely, uniquely designed for me!"

Crystal made a plan. She changed her diet by limiting bread and pasta amounts, she stopped drinking alcohol completely and she started to look at salads and plant based proteins.

HORSE	RIDER	CENTAURED
PILATES CLASSES TWICE WEEKLY	DEVELOPED SELF DISCIPLINE	BEGAN ART CLASSES
WALKED 7KM TO WORK AND HOME	DEVELOPED ROUTINES	ENERGY LEVELS GLOWED
YOGA TWICE WEEKLY	SELF RESPONSIBILITY GREW	FELT SENSUOUS
CHANGED DIET COMPLETELY	STOPPED PARTYING	CONSCIOUSNESS IN MOMENT GREW
INCREASED SLEEP	STOPPED COMPARING SELF	HAPPINESS IN ACHIEVEMENTS
PLANNING WEIGHTS WORKOUTS	DEVELOPED FAITH IN PROCESS	SELF ACCEPTANCE AND RESPECT
BEGAN TEACHING PILATES	COURAGE TO BELIEVE IN SELF	GRATITUDE

Wisdom of the ages a call to arms, longevity of being over 40 years old.
You are never too old to be young!

"If you can't fly, then run,
If you can't run, then walk,
If you can't walk, then crawl
But whatever you do
You have to keep moving forward!" Martin Luther King Jr.

We are alive on this blue marble much longer now than previously ever thought possible. In the early 1900's the life expectancy of men and women was fifty, in the industrialised regions of the world. Obviously it is a lot longer now, and eighty is no longer thought of as an unusual age. We expect to live longer, and some of us are going for posterity! However, we have to be careful about what we wish for. As someone who has spent a lot of time communing with older individuals, it seems to me that it take a great deal of courage to make the decision to take charge of our health choices. At times it is a battle of will to overcome a youth focused society and I have often been prescribed to, with what being over 50 means, and it is not pretty even though I have none of the symptoms described! A general perception of ageing as entailing a loss of strength and stature pervades. My contention is that rather, we are the wiser warriors for our experiences of life, who can maintain our psychophysiology as long as possible. We are flexible thinkers who have survived and succeeded in our many tasks and we have experienced all kinds of adversities. Our ability to teach our horse new tricks is worth fighting for, worth grasping in both hands and worth working every angle!

Gravity

The longer we are in this psychophysiological state we have to contest with gravity on all levels and that's really the nub of it, the gravity of our situation. It pushes us down and it is a force to be reckoned with, especially with changes in our physicality being realities to deal with. Our nerves are more vulnerable, our eyesight and hearing changes, and brain functions gives us cause to pause for remembrances, like why didn't I make a shopping list?

We need to actively seek out health for today and tomorrow whatever that may bring. This gives us more opportunities to "be" in our Third Nature and to become stronger in our ability as flexible thinkers, to make adjustments to the sails of our full speed lives.

We can develop a calmer energy using the natural world we belong to as a background.

We can use nature to nurture the energy we do have.

We can encourage our peace of mind, and then find a placement of our self on this planet. By taking the time to actively garden or to visit a garden, a park, the sea or a lake or river; by watching nature at work and play, and understanding that's where we came from and what we are. We become One then with the forests, the sea, the gardens, Nature, and we know that is still our World.

Then we understand that we need to defy gravity and learn to use our mind's eye to fly!

People are not a number, they are everything and every number they have always been. It is a great sum, yes 40 is different to 50 is different to 60,70,80,90,100, but do these numbers mean we?

This book has partially been a discovery that every person you have ever been, from your conception, through your infant hood, childhood, teens and adulthood is still very much alive within you right now.

All of you Live until you Die!

Holding on to health at any age is possible, it takes modifications and fortitude each day. It is a choice to pick up the reins and ride, a commitment to be strong on all levels. Every time we pick up the weight of ourselves and fight against gravity we grow a bit more, we meet the foe of negativity head on, and our independence to live on our own terms is won.

We will not be 10, 20, or 30 years old again, but we have not lost those numbers. They are still a part of who we are and make up part of the best we can be now, in this conscious moment. We are the legends that our younger peers look up to because we lived long, prospered and are still moving forwards.

Making Fun of Movement

The lighthearted look at life makes use of Third Nature energy to change mood states, and there are even laughter clinics, in some healing centres. All through this book we have used cartoons to capture the quirky side of our nature, and I believe that humour is a powerful tool from our higher thought defenses, and employing it without harm to others, taps into enjoyable moments shared or alone.

We are most motivated in movement by fun leading to laughter, which is in itself, a whole body exercise. Watching and being involved with people at play, leads us to a feeling of lightness of life in that moment. Children's best games as we have seen, involve as much laugher and excitement as possible! They throw themselves into the joy of it literally.

It's no surprise that comedy shows are some of the most popular and longest running television shows because they use the key of "funny" to open the door of smiling relaxed interest. If we can join in on a game or an activity, that gives us the opportunity to exercise our smiling and laughter muscles, which in turn employs our higher thought processes, even the darkest spaces can have light! For it is in those conscious moments, that we can leave the mundane behind, forget the blasé, and elevate the monotony of an everyday rote to find ourselves Centaured in a conscious moment of a created harmony.

This is a refreshment of the psychophysiological, it washes out negative energy states and gives us an opportunity to see situations from a more positive perspective.

CHART OF THREE
THE TRINITY OF THREE

ᛘ	ᛉ	ᚹ
RIDER	HORSE	CENTAUR
FIRST NATURE	SECOND NATURE	THIRD NATURE
INSIGHT	HINDSIGHT	FORESIGHT
PSYCHOLOGICAL	PHYSIOLOGICAL	PSYCHOPHYSIOLOGICAL
MOTIVATION	ACTIVATION	CONSOLIDATION
MIND	BODY	PSYCHOSOMA
CONSUMER ITEMS MONEY	FOOD	LOVE
SLIPS BETWEEN TIME	STUCK IN THE TEMPORAL	COMPLETELY ATEMPORAL

Caterpillars and all their Concerns.....

It was easy enough to wiggle along.
Calculus C.C. Made a great study of each
stem he traversed.
Yes, he could get a wiggle on with the best
of em!
He knew red when he saw it! Straight
under the nearest leaf, or flat up
against the dark bark of stem as
still as a stove pipe... all blended
together... the perfect disguise against
danger; well, almost.
His caterpillar colleagues whose quickness
of spirit did not quite match his own,
often disappeared from the forest of
shrubbery - never to be seen again!

And so the life of wiggle, eat and hide
moved apace with the waxing and waning
of each new day.
This day Calculus C.C began with a rattle
in his wiggle! It was an unnerving
anxious anxiety.
He moved forward trembling; backwards
→

wobbling, and all his legs locked about the leaf he shook upon.

"I can't wiggle, I can't move, I am undone!"
Shaking calamity comes to caterpillars in anxious moments. Calculus C.C knew this well.
He began to spin in a dizzying rush to escape.
The more he spun, the tighter the net of nervous tension held him!
There was no up, no down, just round and around and around!
"Help" he cried, from deep inside this tunnel; this tied terror taking over.
Blackness blocked the light of the sun and brought what seemed eternal night.
Calculus C.C stopped screaming. Crying, he sat, paused and defeated-(devoid of any!)- despairing of any hope of a wiggle, except perhaps wigor mortis...
Days waxed and waned ... a star appeared, an aperture of light!
Calculus C.C saw it... he stretched for it, he put his shoulder back and breathed, then he reached →

143

towards it. A crack, a set of stars, white light; Calculus C.C's eyes were lit with suns. He stretched and moved forward, inch by inch... he pushed forward!
A great burst of colour came upon him and he stretched.. WINGS!
Who knew that from those beginning wiggles great things would grow?
All the suffering, all the darkness and still, an anxious caterpillar has the potential for FLIGHT!

REFERENCES

Introduction

Page 10:   Rachel McLish, Cover Muscle and Fitness, April 1982.
Page 10:   Arnold Schwarzenegger, won Mr Universe aged only 20 and then went on to win Mr Olympia seven times.
Page 12:   John Bowlby; noted British psychologist, psychiatrist and psychoanalyst who made enormous contributions to the study and knowledge of child development and especially attachment theory.

Chapter 1

Page 15:   Sigmund Freud; Austrian born and the founder of psychoanalysis and possibly the most influential thinker within mental health. Citations will all be found within his Collected Works which span many volumes.
Page 15:   Irvin Yalom; "Staring at the Sun", 2008, Angus & Robertson.
Page 17:   Albert Einstein; German born scientist who proposed so much of theoretical physics it's hard to begin to describe. Quote attributed to: Roger Sessions on January 8, 1950 titled "How a 'Difficult' Composer Gets That Way", and it included a version of the saying attributed to Einstein [AERS]: I also remember a remark of Albert Einstein, which certainly applies to music. He said, in effect, that everything should be as simple as it can be but not simpler!
Page 18:   Eric Berne; Canadian psychiatrist who devised Transactional Analysis and wrote "Games People Play."
Page 19:   Abraham Maslow; American psychologist who proposed "Maslow's Hierarchy of Needs."
Page 20:   Rollo May; American psychologist specialising in existential psychotherapy.
Page 21:   Donald Winnicott; English paediatrician and child psychiatrist hugely contributed to Object Relations Theory.
Page 21:   Margaret Mahler; Hungarian physician and psychoanalysis who devised child separation individuation theory.
Page 21:   John Bowlby; ibid.
Page 21:   Konrad Lorenz; Austrian Zoologist and 1973 Nobel Prize winner.
Page 21:   John Watson; American psychologist who established the School of Behaviourism, 1913.
Page 21:   B.F. Skinner; American Psychologist who devised Operant Conditioning.
Page 21:   Martin Seligman; American psychologist who has popularised Positive Psychology.
Page 25:   Sigmund Freud, ibid.
Page 25:   Harry Potter; fictional character from the phenomenally successful books and movies written by J.K.Rowling.

Chapter 2

Page 31:   Abraham Maslow, ibid.

www.ingramcontent.com/pod-product-compliance
Lightning Source LLC
Chambersburg PA
CBHW051617030426
42334CB00030B/3230